EVERYTHING Y
TO FIND OUT IF YOU
AND BEGIN THE RIG

... NOW.

Q: Can any medicine cause an allergic reaction?

Q: What will happen if my child's rhinitis (hay fever) condition is allowed to go medically untreated?

Q: My child is coughing and wheezing. How do I know if an allergy is the cause?

Q: How can I tell which brand of anti-asthma medication is right for my child?

Dr. Robert Feldman has successfully treated thousands of children for allergy conditions caused by food, medicine, pollen, household products, and other agents. In this sourcebook he answers all your allergy questions with clear, specific information, personal case histories, and prescription charts, including:

- A seasonal, pollen calendar for every area of the country
- Complete lists of brand-name medicines and how they should be administered to your child
- Cautions on unproven, controversial, and experimental allergy treatments
- Comprehensive lists of foods and substances that can trigger allergic reactions.

"Details the major types of allergic conditions that plague children and explains how parents can best communicate with their child's physicians in monitoring the child's ailment to relieve symptoms."
—SciTech Book News

"The best book in a crowded field."   *—Medical Self Care*

"A comprehensive guide . . . provides a practical foundation for the layperson and has an excellent resource section . . . has been on our recommended reading list for over a year!"
—Mothers of Asthmatics, Inc.

B. ROBERT FELDMAN, M.D., is Associate Attending Physician, Division of Pediatric Allergy, Columbia-Presbyterian Medical Center, and Assistant Clinical Professor of Pediatrics at Columbia College of Physicians and Surgeons, both in New York City.

DAVID CARROLL is the author of more than a dozen books, including *The Complete Book of Natural Medicines*.

THE COMPLETE BOOK OF CHILDREN'S ALLERGIES

B. ROBERT FELDMAN, M.D.

with DAVID CARROLL

WARNER BOOKS

A Warner Communications Company

The advice in this book can be a valuable addition
to the advice of your child's doctor, and is designed for
your use under his or her care and direction.

Warner Books Edition

This Warner Books edition is published by arrangement with Times Books

Warner Books, Inc., 666 Fifth Avenue, New York, NY 10103

 A Warner Communications Company

Printed in the United States of America
First Warner Books Printing: June 1989
10 9 8 7 6 5 4 3 2

Library of Congress Cataloging-in-Publication Data

Feldman, B. Robert
  The complete book of children's allergies.
  Includes index.
  1. Pediatric allergy—Popular works. I. Carroll,
David, 1942- . II. Title. [DNLM: 1. Hypersensitivity—in
infancy & childhood—popular works. WD 300 F312c]
RJ386.F45 1986   618.92′97   86-1354
ISBN 0-446-38765-7 (pbk.)

To my wife, Clare, who provided constant encouragement, my children David and Janet, who knew that eventually it would be completed, and finally in loving memory of my parents: Morris and Florence Feldman.

—B.R.F.

Acknowledgments

First, let me acknowledge the unknowing contribution of all the patients I have cared for during the past twenty-two years. Their constant questions provided me with the incentive to think about and eventually to write this book.

My sincere appreciation to my close friend and colleague, William J. Davis, M.D., director of the Allergy Division, Babies Hospital, Columbia-Presbyterian Medical Center, and to my long-time associate, Charles H. Feldman, M.D., for reviewing the manuscript and providing me with their constructive criticism.

Finally, to my co-author, David Carroll, who with his literary talent has left his indelible imprint on this book, I extend my thanks for a difficult job well done.

—B.R.F.

Contents

Part One

An Introduction to Allergy

About Allergy

It's estimated that in the United States today 30 to 40 million people suffer from some kind of allergic condition. Many of your friends are no doubt numbered among them, and if you are a member of this not-so-exclusive club your child probably is too, for allergic tendencies can be inherited. But first things first.

If your child is an allergy sufferer, you already know all you care to concerning the symptoms this difficult malady brings: the sneezing, the wheezing, the all-night bouts with the vaporizer. There is, however, an invisible mechanism that works behind these outward signs which is little understood even by many long-time allergy sufferers. Let us examine what triggers this common, familiar, yet basically mysterious quirk of the human machine.

What Is an Allergy?

There are many ways to define allergy, most of them unduly technical. For our purposes an allergy is simply an abnormal response of the body to a substance that is ordinarily harmless for most people. Ragweed is a good case in point. Invite ten of your friends to a picnic. Place them in front of a flowering plant and ask them to inhale. Of the group, six or seven will probably be unaffected. One or two will start to sneeze within minutes—some lightly, some with gusto —and one may have an all-out allergic attack. The meaning of this scene is that most people who are exposed to ragweed pollen will not react at all, but those of us who are allergic to this substance can and will exhibit a variety of symptoms.

The skin, nose and lungs are the parts of the body most commonly involved during an allergic episode—the section of the body where the allergic attack takes place is called the shock organ—though the list of organs which may possibly come under siege does not stop here. It includes:

the nose (hay fever)
the lungs (asthma)

the skin (rashes)
the eyes (allergic conjunctivitis)
the stomach (food sensitivities)
the ears (fluid behind the eardrum)
the head (headaches and sinus troubles)

Allergic symptoms may involve a single part of the body, as the lungs in asthma or the skin in atopic dermatitis. In some conditions such as hay fever, the eyes and nose will be involved, and in anaphylaxis, which is a generalized form of allergic reaction, the lungs, skin, central nervous system, and heart will take part in the response.

Allergens and Antibodies

When does an allergic reaction begin? Basically, it starts the moment a child comes in contact with a foreign substance known as an allergen or antigen (though not exactly synonymous, the two terms are often used interchangeably), and becomes sensitized to this allergen. Antigens are foreign substances (proteins and polysaccharides) that can cause an immune response in any person. An allergen is a type of antigen that is capable of causing symptoms in an allergic individual.

We will take a closer look at the allergic mechanism in a following section, but at this point it is necessary only to know that for a sensitized person, allergens are the triggers of allergic episodes, and that they include an incredibly wide spectrum of possible substances ranging from apples to zucchini. The most common offenders include pollen from trees, grasses and weeds as well as molds, dust, foods, industrial pollutants, animal dander, insect stings, and household chemicals such as detergents or perfumes. The most frequent allergies plaguing children are hay fever and bronchial asthma, followed by skin conditions such as hives or atopic dermatitis, sensitivities to such common foods as nuts or dairy products, and reactions to stinging insects.

It is interesting to realize that different children who are sensitive to the same allergen may respond to this substance with totally different clinical symptoms. Whereas five-year-old Brian develops a runny nose and tearing eyes during the ragweed season, nine-year-old Alice wheezes whenever she is exposed to this common weed. Why such varying organ system involvement occurs in reaction to the same allergen is not clearly understood.

Potential allergy-causing substances are thus in our environment every hour of the night and day, whether we are aware of them or not. They enter the human system via four main "doors":

In the substances we eat: these are called ingestants. Almost any food or drug you can think of may be included, along with an ever-growing number of chemical compounds added to our foods.

In the materials we touch: these are called contactants. Poison ivy is a prime example.

In the chemicals injected into our bodies: injected materials. These include medicines such as penicillin and insulin.

In substances which we inhale: inhalants. While pollen grains are the most common offenders, industrial and household pollutants are substances to be reckoned with.

Most children will not develop signs or symptoms of allergy regardless of the number of allergens to which they are exposed. However, for approximately 10 to 20 percent of children, contact with these otherwise harmless allergens will trigger an allergic response. Why one child develops this type of reaction and a sibling or the child next door fails to react in a similar manner is not completely understood. Nevertheless, we do have the answers for many of the questions asked about why allergies begin.

It's in Your Genes

We know, for example, that when a child's parents or grandparents are allergic, the chances of that child developing allergic symptoms are greater than those of a child born to a nonallergic family. On a statistical basis, though exact numbers are difficult to obtain, approximately 10 to 20 percent of all children in the United States will develop some kind of allergic problem. Those youngsters with one allergic parent will have about a 30 to 35 percent chance of joining the ranks of the allergic, and if both parents are allergic, the possibility jumps to 50 or 60 percent, more than one out of two. If there is absolutely no history of allergy in a child's background, he or she still has about a one out of six chance of developing an allergy. So the end result is that while a family history of sensitivity is usually but not *inevitably* a ticket to allergy, neither does lack of it in the family background guarantee immunity.

While there is a strong genetic tendency toward allergy among certain children, *specific sensitivities* are not inherited. It is the *potential* to develop allergy that is passed on from parent to child, not a particular allergic condition.

Take, for example, a young mother named Elisabeth who is sensitive to dogs and cats. Her son Stephen is also born with allergies, but his attacks are set off by grass and ragweed. Another mother, Valerie, has two children, a boy and a girl. Both children are allergic, but their reactions differ not only from each other but also from their mother. Valerie's son sneezes when he is exposed to feathers, and her daughter develops a rash whenever she drinks milk. Valerie herself has asthma. Moreover, even if a parent has an especially severe allergy, the children will not necessarily develop either this particular allergy *or* its particular intensity—neither specific sensitivity nor degree of seriousness is inherited.

At What Age Do Allergic Symptoms Usually Develop?

The time it takes for a person to become sensitized to a specific allergen can vary from months to decades. Why is it that a person can be exposed over and over again for many years to the same allergen and then, on a certain hour of a certain day, seemingly out of the blue, have a reaction to it? No one knows. But this is how the process works. The common notion that if you did not have hay fever as a child you will never get it as an adult is a myth.

I know, for example, of one twenty-nine-year-old woman who rarely sneezed. On a cross-country driving trip she and her husband stopped to camp somewhere in the deserts of New Mexico, a region to which, ironically, many people with allergies migrate in order to escape the pollens that proliferate in the damper, greener areas back east. The next morning the woman awoke, sat up in her sleeping bag, stretched, and started to sneeze. She proceeded to sneeze her way through Arizona, into Nevada, across California, on into Oregon and Washington, then most of the way home to New York; and to my knowledge she is still sneezing somewhere today. This woman was carrying around a potential sensitivity to a particular antigen for many years, perhaps most of her life. One day that potential became actual.

Yet here's the rub. While allergies may develop at any age in a person's lifetime, there is a greater tendency—a *far* greater tendency—for them to start up during childhood. Why? Partly because a child's immune system is more active and sensitive than an adult's. This means that not only are school-age children more likely than adults to acquire allergies, but so are infants, even the youngest. Indeed, the various digestive problems and skin rashes infants develop in the first months of life may be the result of allergic reactions to their diet. New parents should be aware that certain symptoms in newborns such as nasal stuffiness, chronic cough, and extreme irritability may ultimately be traced to allergic causes.

It All Starts in the Immune System

The main function of the immune system is to defend the body against invasion by bacteria, viruses, and assorted troublemaking foreign substances; also to eliminate any abnormal cells within the body that are potentially cancerous. During the course of our lifetime, millions and millions of these antigens enter our bodies; as you are reading this paragraph, numbers of them are entering your system and being processed by your immune system, pounced on and eliminated. People in whom this immune surveillance system is not working properly, such as those with AIDS, become ready targets of practically any unfriendly bacteria, often succumbing to germs which to a healthy immune mechanism would present nothing more challenging than a routine house-cleaning job.

The immune system is the principal defense force of the body. The various components of this system are scattered throughout the body. Collectively, the thymus gland, spleen, tonsils, adenoids, lymph nodes (especially those located in the intestinal tract), and bone marrow are the main parts of this "system." The cells that are the front-line fighters of this protective system are special white blood cells called lymphocytes.

Lymphocytes are produced in the bone marrow and then mature in either the thymus gland or the lymphoid tissue of the intestinal tract. These lymphocytes have special abilities and are able to protect you and me against bacteria, viruses, and cancerous cells.

What characterizes the sensitization process? When a child has become sensitized, it means that a specific type of white blood cell within his or her system, called a plasma cell, has been stimulated to produce a special protein known as an antibody. These antibodies circulate freely throughout the child's body; when they happen to meet with certain foreign substances which have entered the body—that is, when they come in contact with allergens—an *allergic* reaction results. This response in turn takes place on the surface of another type of white blood cell called a mast cell. During the reaction the mast cells release a relatively large number of chemical compounds collectively called mediators; the best known of these is histamine, the chemical culprit responsible for most of the sneezing, teary eyes and sniffling that exasperate some 20 to 25 million of us every year.

How many lymphocytes are there in your body right now? While precise counts are impossible to make, there are probably at any given time about a trillion lymphocytes in the human organism capable of producing another million trillion antibodies. Indeed, in the time it has taken you to read this page your body has already produced millions of antibody molecules, each one unique, like snowflakes.

Each time your child is exposed to a new antigen, be it a food, virus or pollen grain, a group of these special antibodies are produced to confront this *specific* foreign substance and react with it. When substance A enters your body, your immune system produces antibodies specially engineered to deal with substance A; when substance B arrives, a new group of antibodies are created to deal exclusively with substance B, and so on. Our protective system —our immunological police force, if you will—is our main line of defense against all invaders from the outer world.

In a healthy child the immunological police force is on duty twenty-four hours a day, ever on the lookout for invaders. Ordinarily the outcome between an antigen and its specific antibody is a foregone conclusion, with the antibody neatly besting the offending substance and routinely removing it. But in the case of an allergy something goes awry: the immune system becomes more of a problem than the foreign object it is attacking—usually nothing more than a harmless pollen or an innocuous food substance—and ends up provoking symptoms worse than anything these innocent substances might cause in a nonsensitized individual. Instead of blocking the development of symptoms, the immune system causes them. Antibodies are produced that do not protect the body. They actually have the opposite effect, serving as the triggers of allergic symptoms. An allergic reaction is, in brief, a protective mechanism gone haywire.

Why Can't Johnny Breathe?

Watch what happens during the course of a normal immune response. Assume, for example, that Billy, age four, has just started nursery school. In his second week in this "public" environment he is exposed to virus A, causing him to develop an upper respiratory infection. Because Billy is in good health, his immune system easily deals with the virus and he recovers within four or five days.

Billy has now been exposed to virus A and his immunological lines of defense have produced antibodies against it. Next time virus A enters Billy's system, his immune system will "remember" that it was once in contact with this bug, and it will produce large numbers of antibodies to block or blunt the virus from causing another respiratory infection.

Fine. Now, take the same child again. This time, though, Billy is experiencing an allergic reaction. See how his immune response misbehaves.

At first the same immunological sequence follows as with virus A. An allergen—in this case a pollen grain—lands on the mucous membrane inside Billy's nose. Blood cells called macrophages present in nearby nasal tissues take this grain, process it, "show" it to the lymphocytes, which then produce antibodies to get rid of it.

The particular antibodies now produced, however, especially in a susceptible, genetically primed child like Billy, are of a special class. They are called *IgE immunoglobulins.*

Ordinarily nonallergic children have very low levels of IgE immunoglobulin antibodies in their bloodstream and are not affected by them. Children reactive to a particular allergen, however, will begin producing IgE antibodies in great abundance whenever they come in contact with this allergen. As these antibodies proliferate, they attach themselves to the surface of certain white blood cells, called basophil cells, which live in the bloodstream, and to mast cells, which are primarily located within the body tissues. Once this process occurs, these mast and basophil cells are said to be "sensitized," and henceforth when exposed to the specific allergen both will become the site of an allergic response.

Now mast cells and basophils are filled with many dense granules throughout their cellular substance, each granule enclosed by a membrane which insulates its chemical compounds from the rest of the cell. These chemical compounds are known as mediators.

Most mediators have chemical names unfamiliar to the layman. There is one which you're probably quite familiar with if there is allergy in your family. It is called histamine, and it is responsible for many of the common symptoms plaguing allergy sufferers. This troublesome chemical is released from the granules when the interaction just discussed takes place between IgE antibodies and the allergen. Once released, it seeps into surrounding local tissues and blood vessels, where it causes swelling and congestion, triggering the maddening itching sensations associated with skin allergies. In the lungs, histamine will narrow the breathing passages, sometimes throwing the victim into a full-fledged asthmatic spasm. In the nose it may cause nasal mucus glands to spew out a watery discharge; in the eyes it produces swollen lids and stinging tears; in the head it will stimulate headaches and sinus congestion; in the stomach, cramps and diarrhea may occur. The more histamine there is in a particular area, the more acute the allergic reaction becomes. It's no fun.

Thus the bare mechanics of allergy. In a mild reaction the symptoms can be controlled with nothing stronger than an over-the-counter antihistamine (note: *anti*histamine). In other situations allergic reactions take a more serious turn, especially when breathing is impaired or skin rashes get out of hand. At such times a physician's help is decidedly in order.

Visiting the Doctor

Identifying Your Child's Symptoms

A runny nose, eyes that tear, a throat that's sore, all may be due to hay fever. Or they may stem from a cold; the symptoms are almost identical. A breathing problem is the result of pollen sensitivity. Or is it a more serious disease? Or then again, perhaps it's just lingering bronchitis. The whole area of symptoms can get downright confusing, especially when many of these disparate symptoms appear simultaneously. How do you as a parent decide whether or not an allergy is behind it all?

Parents can make several valuable clinical observations when the question of allergic involvement arises. Short of a doctor's analysis, they are among the most efficient diagnostic resources a parent can know about.

Start by looking for *repeating patterns of symptoms* (listed below) *that tend to occur at regular intervals,* especially during specific months or seasons. Spring and fall are the most likely times for such patterns to surface. They can, however, come at any time, cold or hot, rain or shine.

Then look for a pattern of symptoms that repeat under identical circumstances. For example, each time young Barbara eats a slice of bread, she starts to wheeze. This should cast suspicion on wheat. Every time Tom stretches out on his down-stuffed quilt, he sneezes. This may indicate an allergy to feathers.

Several years ago a young married couple and their five-year-old daughter moved from a small city in Iran to Boston. Within several months the child began to have regular sneezing bouts and to develop skin rashes, something she had never done before. The parents noted that the child's rash worsened after trips to a local playground. Following careful observation the parents discovered that their daughter's reaction was caused by contact with dogs. As it happened, the child had grown up in a town without dogs of any kind. In the United States, her five-year-old heart became enchanted by the friendly creatures, so much so that she ran up and embraced every one that happened by her on the playground. This frequent contact caused her to become sensitized to the animal's dander, and soon after her symptoms appeared. This girl had the potential to react allergically to dogs, but the symptoms did not become apparent until she had repeated exposure to them.

Look for a set pattern of symptoms such as sneezing, nasal congestion or cough that becomes *chronic.* Be suspicious of a cold that drags on month after month; it probably isn't a cold at all. Or a cough that won't go away, or an annoying, itchy, persistent rash. Generally speaking, a viral or bacterial infection rarely lasts more than one or two weeks at a time, maximum; an allergy can go on for months or even years. If coldlike symptoms continue for five or six weeks, such lingering discomfort should put you on guard. More than likely you're looking at an allergic response.

What exactly are allergic symptoms? Though I will, of course, go into this question in some detail when examining the various specific allergic conditions in the sections that follow, a brief run-through here of the most common symptoms, taken organ by organ, will help you make your observations more quickly.

The Most Common Allergic Symptoms

The skin: An allergic reaction involving the skin typically appears as a rash that is almost always very itchy. There is no consistent appearance for such an allergic rash. Anything from a red raised wheal, a typical hive, to the raw, oozing, reddened rash of acute eczema can result from an allergic reponse.

The eyes: Symptoms include redness of the conjunctiva (the white portion of the eye), tearing and itching, swelling of the upper and lower lids, and the production of a gelatinous mucus secretion.

The nose: Foremost, of course, is the runny nose. How to tell if it's from an allergy or a cold? One clue is that the nasal discharge caused by an allergy has a thin, clear, watery consistency, while the discharge from a cold or flu is thick, whitish, and heavy. A second observation is that even though children run about for weeks on end with a leaking nose, if the symptom is from an allergy the child will generally *not* develop an irritation of the upper lip and the nostrils, while children suffering from a viral or bacteria-caused nasal drip will.

Another important nasal symptom is sneezing. The child will tell you that there seems to be something blocking his nose. He can't smell very well or breathe through his nose. If a child sniffs constantly and wipes his nose with a passion, sometimes so frequently that the skin becomes raw, chances are he's allergic.

The mouth: Look for complaints that the top (roof) of the mouth itches and futile attempts to use the tongue in order to get relief from this maddening symptom. There are also complaints of a sensation that something is constantly dripping down the back of the throat. This is called a postnasal drip.

The ears: Allergic symptoms include a sensation of dripping within the ear, of itchiness, or of a feeling that the ears are clogged. A pre-speech child may tug on her earlobes, rub the side of her head, or frequently cock her head to one side. A child who can talk may tell you that she seems to hear things "through water"—which is almost the case. At times the external portions of the ear may become reddened. Infants with hearing difficulties due to allergy will often show signs of language development problems. They may be late talkers, if they talk much at all, and you may notice that they have trouble relating easily with their peers.

The chest: Watch for recurrent cough unassociated with other signs of a cold. There may be shortness of breath and an inability to take a deep breath. Also, a sensation of tightness in the chest accompanied by a whistling wheeze heard most often when the child is breathing out is the most typical symptom of asthma. The child may also complain of a pain in the chest, usually associated with prolonged coughing or when taking a deep breath. This pain is caused by stretching the muscles between the ribs and is common during an asthma attack.

The gastrointestinal tract: The most frequent symptoms consist of nausea, vomiting and diarrhea. A child who is having an asthma attack may complain of abdominal pain, which is caused by the diaphragm being forced downward onto the stomach. When a young child has an asthma attack, he may swallow large amounts of air, resulting in distension of and pain in the stomach.

Generalized allergic response: An allergic reaction does not always occur in only one area. It may strike many parts of the body simultaneously in the form of a *generalized* response or, as it is known technically, anaphylaxis. Anaphylaxis is caused by a massive release of chemical mediators in many organ systems *all at the same time* with possible involvement of the lungs (wheezing, breathing difficulties), skin (generalized hives and swelling), intestinal tract (vomiting, diarrhea) and the vascular system (drop in blood pressure with possible loss of consciousness). In other words, practically the entire body is affected. When a severe generalized reaction occurs, waste no time—*the outcome can be fatal if the condition is not given immediate medical attention.*

When Should You Visit the Doctor?

When does an allergic problem become serious enough to warrant a trip to the doctor? This depends on two basic factors: the *frequency* of the child's symptoms and their *severity.*

Though it's difficult to make absolute recommendations, a good rule of thumb is this: if a child's symptoms can be controlled by using over-the-counter antiallergic drugs such as antihistamines and decongestants, then no additional medical consultation may be necessary. If these drugs do not work, then a doctor should be consulted. If the symptoms are worsening, either in duration or in severity, stop medicating the child yourself and get the immediate advice of a physician.

General Practitioner or Allergist?

Sometimes, of course, parents suspect their child's problem is an allergic one but do not know for certain. In this case a visit to the family doctor to discuss the situation is certainly appropriate. If the family physician can relieve the child's symptoms with medication, which is often the case, then a trip to the specialist is unnecessary. Most allergy problems in this country are not treated by allergists. Of the 30 to 40 million allergy sufferers in this country, the treatment of most is quite well managed by the family physician.

In some cases, however, the child's allergic problem will prove to be complicated or difficult. The primary physician may then feel it's necessary to turn the case over to someone specially trained in this area of medicine. Enter the allergist.

An allergist is an M.D. who has undergone a period of specialized training in the recognition, evaluation and treatment of clinical allergy and immunology problems. A referral to his office usually is indicated when your child's symptoms are not responding to the treatment recommended by the family physician, or the allergic symptoms persist and actually seem to be increasing in intensity.

In other words, if your child is experiencing continual or worsening symptoms, I feel it is appropriate to visit an allergist for a consultation. If there is an ongoing problem, I do not feel it is wise to wait on the chancy grounds that your child may "outgrow" the condition. I have definite reservations concerning any physician who assures parents that their child will outgrow his or her allergy. If there is no obvious improvement of your child's suspected problem, you should take it upon yourself to at the very least get a second medical opinion. While it is certainly true that many young children with significant allergy problems will lose their symptoms as they grow older, I certainly don't know how to predict who will be the lucky ones, and I have yet to meet the physician who has the ability to see into the future!

Finding the Right Allergist

Though there are many ways to find an allergist, perhaps the most reliable is by referral from your own physician. Chances are your doctor has worked with this specialist in the past and that they maintain a good relationship with each other. This is an important factor. Occasionally parents of an allergic child will find themselves caught between the conflicting opinions of two professionals. Your pediatrician feels that each time a child has a bout of asthma an antibiotic should be used; your allergist believes there is good reason to withhold this medicine. The parent and of course the child then become pawns in what sometimes turns into a tense, unpleasant situation, one that could have been avoided had the physician and specialist chosen each other at the beginning. Remember, simply because you are referred to a specialist does not mean your regular physician will be removed from the scene. Your primary physician and your allergist *must* be able to work together if your child is to get the care he or she deserves.

If for some reason your doctor is hesitant to give you a referral—occasionally some doctors will feel slighted when one is requested—you can contact the local medical societies in your area and request a list of board-certified allergists. Board-certified means that a doctor has successfully completed a course of training in the area of allergic medicine, and that he or she has passed specific examinations in this field. While board certification is obviously no guarantee that this person will prove to be the best doctor for your child, it at least assures you that this individual has had the proper training and experience.

If you live in an area with a medical school nearby, you can also call the school's information center or referral service and inquire concerning allergists affiliated with their staff. In general you can assume that doctors associated with an accredited medical school will be particularly well qualified. They make a point of keeping up with what's new and are continually being exposed to the latest advances in their fields.

Finally, check with your friends, neighbors and relatives. Word of mouth is still one of the best ways of finding what you're looking for.

What Does an Allergist Do?

At the initial visit an allergist will require a highly detailed history of the child's present symptoms and medical past. This personal evaluation is the single most important diagnostic tool in the allergist's arsenal. All that is up-to-date and miraculous in modern laboratory technology is not worth the paper this page is printed on unless it comes coupled with a thorough description of your child's physical, social and psychological past. And you as parent are responsible for this description. The better organized this history is, the more detailed and complete, the more it will help your child.

After the child's detailed history is taken—more on this below—a complete physical examination is made, followed by medical tests when appropriate. These tests may run the gamut from a simple blood sample to sophisticated X-ray studies with many, many possibilities in between. We will look at some of the more common tests below.

After all this input—the history, the physical examination, and the laboratory evaluation—has been weighed and considered, the doctor will make the final diagnosis of the child's condition and outline an appropriate program of treatment. In some cases a limited course of medication to control symptoms is all that is required. In others a variety of treatments will be called for including allergy injections, dietary manipulation, environmental control measures and special prescription medicines. The thoughtful allergist will design a treatment program for your child that provides him with the maximum medical benefit and yet does not place an undue economic or logistical burden on the patient and family.

Preparing for the First Visit to an Allergist

Bear in mind that a good allergist or pediatrician will insist on including both parent(s) and child as integral parts of the physician-parent-patient triangle. This relationship is the cornerstone of a successful partnership and will be crucial in guaranteeing the best possible results. Many chronic allergic conditions necessitate a long-term ongoing relationship between physician and family. This relationship must be founded on the concept that while the doctor is the coach, everyone is an important part of the team. It must by no means be orchestrated by an aloof autocrat who sits behind a mahogany desk, writing mysterious prescriptions and issuing orders. If the physician you're seeing never seems to have enough time for you, if he doesn't encourage your questions or if he answers the ones you manage to slip in with condescension or, worse, unintelligible "doctorese," then you're probably involved with the wrong person. Consider looking elsewhere before a formal long-term commitment is made.

At the same time, parents must play their part, too. Those who are not taking the time to formulate important questions before they visit their physician are not doing their job. Those who allow the doctor to do all the talking and all the thinking, who fail to keep a watchful eye on their child's condition at home and who do not consider themselves as a fundamental part of the healing unit are missing an important opportunity to help everyone involved. What is most important in the doctor-patient-parent partnership is the free flow of ideas, the sharing of observations, and a mutual commitment to the patient. If one partner remains uninvolved, the whole therapeutic program automatically fails.

I strongly advise that at your first visit to an allergist you come prepared to participate in all decisions and to share the important facts of your child's past medical history. I suggest that you sit down several days before the first visit, either by yourself, or better, with your spouse, and write down significant facts related to your child's allergic past. The more prepared you are to answer the doctor's questions at the first visit, the more immediate feedback the doctor will be able to give back to you. Here is a checklist of the possible questions the doctor may ask concerning your child's personal allergic history, and to which you should have answers ready.

A Checklist of Your Child's History

- What was the date of the child's first attack?
- What were the specific circumstances involved at the time of this attack? Did the child eat something new, breathe something unusual, rub something exotic on his skin? Was he bitten or stung? If so, by what?

- Where was the child located when the first attack occurred? In the city? The country? At home? On the playground? At the movies? At the house of a friend? In school? At camp?
  - During what time of year were the symptoms noticed?
  - What medical treatment, if any, was provided?
  - What was the apparent outcome of the treatment?
  - How long did this first bout of allergy last?

The question of how the symptoms have evolved since their initial onset will be of key importance in this history:

- How often do the symptoms now occur?
- Do the symptoms tend to appear when the child is in one specific geographic location—in rural areas, in urban areas, at home, by the sea, etc? Does the condition improve when the child travels from one geographic area to another—i.e., from the seashore to the city, from the mountains to the desert, etc.?
- How severe is the attack when it occurs? In what physical and psychological ways does the child react?
- Describe all the symptoms of the suspected allergic response, even those that seem insignificant or secondary. In what part of the body are they predominantly located?
- Is the child's condition presently stable? Does it seem to be getting worse? Is it improving?
- Are there any differences in symptoms during the day and during the night? At what time of day are the symptoms most intense? Is there a specific seasonal pattern to the problem: is it worse during one particular time of year, better during another?

Then the question of diet:

- What in general does the child eat? How closely can you describe your child's average daily menu?
- Do you know of any particular foods that seem to cause allergic symptoms? Which foods are generally disliked? Which ones are most enjoyed and most frequently eaten?
- If the child is thought to be allergic to certain foods, how long does it take for the reaction to set in? Which organs are affected? In what way?
- What drugs were taken during pregnancy? Was the child breast-fed? If not, what formula was used?

Also important is information regarding previous medical consultations and the child's general medical history.

- What medical treatments have been given in the past for allergic symptoms? How long were they taken? Give the specific names of the medicines prescribed, and the doses. (Descriptions such as "a blue pill" or "a clear liquid" are practically worthless. Provide the actual *names* of the medicines, either from the pharmacist who supplied them or the doctor who prescribed them; both parties should have this information on record.)

· Have there been any problems related to the medications?

· Have any prior laboratory tests been made? What were the results? If possible the results from any previous test should be brought to the office at the time of the first visit. Copies or summaries of consultations can be gotten by contacting the original doctor and requesting that he or she forward the records to the new physician's office.

Be prepared to discuss the child's family history:

· What are the parents' occupations? Does the child have brothers and sisters? Do any of them have a history of allergy?

· Is there a record of allergy in the family? (This means not only the father and mother but grandparents, brothers and sisters, even uncles, aunts and cousins.) How badly do any of these family members suffer from this ailment?

· Is there any unusual medical history in the family? Are there other chronic conditions that the doctor should be informed of?

· Have there been unusual family problems that have gone undiagnosed?

· Has the child ever been hospitalized? If so, what for?

· What kind of immunizations have been given in the past?

· What was the mother's pregnancy with the child like? Were there any noteworthy incidents or problems, especially feeding problems, during the first few months of life?

You should also be prepared to describe the immediate environment that presently surrounds your child. This applies especially to your home and all the many things in it:

· How old is your house?

· What kind of heating system do you have? If your heating system is forced air, how often do you change the filters? Do you use humidifiers? Do you have air conditioning?

· Is your basement dry? Damp? Does your child frequent this area very often?

· What are your pillows made of? Your carpets? Your blankets? Does anyone in your home work with strong chemicals such as the paints, glues or photographic substances used by hobbyists? Do you live near any industrial plants?

· Is your child ever exposed to unusual substances at a babysitter's home or play group?

• What about the child's toys? Are they stuffed or fashioned from unusual materials? What objects does the child sleep with at night? Which toys are played with most during the day?

• Do you have a pet in the house? What type? These include the less conspicuous varieties such as birds and hamsters as well as cats and dogs. How much contact does the child have with the animal? How long have you owned it? Have you ever noted any strange reactions on the child's part after the child and the pet have been together for a period of time?

• How dry, dust free and chemical free is the child's room, especially the area where she sleeps? Is there a carpet on the floor? What type of material is the carpet made of? How recently has the room been painted? What type of paint was used?

Parents should come to their first visit with questions of their own. Draw up a list before you arrive. Consider all the many questions you've wondered about through the years concerning your child's condition; jot them down. Some of these questions may be unanswerable on the first visit, and some may never be answerable. But you should ask anything you like, and usually there will be answers.

Briefly, you can hope for all of the following from an allergist's evaluation:

• a decision regarding the allergic or nonallergic cause of your child's symptoms.

• a specific recommendation or plan of treatment for the child's condition. In general, allergies cannot be cured. But with the forms of treatment available today, most can be very well controlled.

• perhaps most important, a sympathetic ear and a dependable source of information that can provide answers from the knowledge of direct experience.

On the other hand, allergists cannot predict the future. Neither at the first meeting nor at any other time can an allergist say with certainty whether a child will get better, get worse or stay the same. He cannot predict whether your child will respond positively to a specific form of treatment or outgrow his symptoms.

What the allergist *can* promise you is that he will provide you with informed, conscientious service and that the most up-to-date and effective methods of modern medicine will be made available to your child. In most cases the combination of these two powerful tools will lead to a successful outcome. In most cases a child can and will be helped.

Evaluating the Allergic Child

Personal History and Physical Exam

Personal history, physical examination, lab tests: of the three the personal history is usually the most important. It should be detailed and very specific. Some physicians request an oral history from parents while others provide a form for the family to fill out at the time of the initial examination or before the first visit to the office. If you are asked to fill out one of these forms, be as thorough as possible. A study of the personal history checklist featured in the preceding chapter will stand you in good stead in this regard.

After the history has been obtained, the doctor will then perform a physical examination of your child. In preparation for this experience, explain to the young person that this part of the visit does not hurt at all. Ever. That it will be more or less like any other examination at any other doctor's office and nothing drastic or bizarre will take place. Height and weight will be checked; the eyes, nose, mouth, and ears will be looked at; the doctor will listen to the heartbeat, examine the skin, take blood pressure, and so on. For the youngest patients it is good psychology to let them touch the medical instruments like the stethoscope or otoscope before the examination begins, to demonstrate their harmlessness. Usually the examination will last no longer than fifteen minutes.

Allergy Tests and How They Work

After the history and physical examination are completed, tests will usually be ordered appropriate to the specific allergic problem. There are, of course, a goodly number of these, the most important of which we will discuss now, close up, from the standpoint of what you should know concerning how these tests work, why they are ordered, what they determine, the ways in which they are administered to the child, the dangers or pain involved, and any other significant facts concerning their operation.

Most allergists' tests are quickly administered and relatively pain-free. Still, it is well within your rights as concerned parent, should you wish it, to request a list of the tests that your child will undergo and to familiarize yourself with it. You can then check this list against the description of allergy tests given below to better understand how they work, and why a certain procedure has been ordered for your child.

A Checklist of Allergy Tests

Blood Tests

Complete Blood Count

PURPOSE   Frequently a complete blood count or CBC will be done to check the overall condition of the blood. A low hemoglobin level indicates that some form of anemia is present. If the white blood cell count is elevated, an infection may be present. This test helps the doctor determine whether the child's symptoms stem from a bacterial/viral infection or from an allergic sensitivity.

FREQUENCY   Standard. It is usually done on the first visit to the doctor and may be repeated at infrequent intervals.

HOW ADMINISTERED   A CBC can be done in two ways. Either by pricking the child's finger and taking a smear, or by removing blood directly via a needle (a process called *venipuncture*). Both methods are usually done by a technician in a laboratory.

PAIN   Both are associated with mild discomfort, though neither is very painful. The venipuncture is probably more menacing, simply because it involves a hypodermic needle.

RESULTS AVAILABLE   In one or two days at most.

Quantitative Immunoglobulins Determination Test

PURPOSE   Here the doctor is looking for three different immunoglobulin proteins: IgG, IgA and IgM (the Ig stands for immunoglobulin). These antibody proteins are normally produced by all of us and are a regular part of the body's immune system. Some children with abnormally low levels of these proteins, specifically IgG, have a tendency to develop severe bacterial infections. Your doctor may suspect that a patient's pattern of repeated infections is associated with such an abnormality, and the gammaglobulin level will give him important information regarding this aspect of the body's defense mechanism. The test will provide evidence of a deficiency of the immune system.

FREQUENCY   Not on a regular basis, generally performed when there is a problem with repeated infections. Usually the test will only be performed once if the results are normal.

HOW ADMINISTERED   By a venipuncture or finger stick. If a child requires both the CBC and a quantitative immunoglobulins test, blood is drawn only once; both tests will then be made from the single sample.

PAIN   Usually mild and momentary when performed by a skilled technician or physician.

RESULTS AVAILABLE   In several days to a week.

Serum IgE Level Determination

PURPOSE   Done quite frequently today, an IgE level determination, like the quantitative immunoglobulins determination test, searches for a specific immunoglobulin protein in the blood—in this case the IgE protein. IgE was first discovered in 1967 and has since been found to be a specific marker for the presence of allergic disease. While an elevation of the IgE in the blood does not invariably accompany allergy problems, approximately 60 to 70 percent of people who have allergic symptoms will also have an increased IgE level, and that's a pretty fair percentage. Examining a blood sample from this perspective, a doctor can thus come to a more definitive conclusion concerning symptoms which look suspiciously like allergy—runny nose, sneezing, etc.—but which can also stem from non-allergic causes.

FREQUENCY   A standard allergy test.

HOW ADMINISTERED   Through venipuncture.

PAIN   Momentary discomfort.

RESULTS AVAILABLE   In several days.

COMMENTS   The IgE will not tell the doctor specifically *what* the person is allergic to, only that with an elevated IgE level there is a very good chance the person *is* allergic. Almost all persons suffering from atopic dermatitis will have a high IgE level.

X-Rays

Conventional X-Ray Study

VARIETIES   The physician may request a number of X-ray studies. Here are the four most common ones.

  • Chest X-ray taken from the back and the side, called PA and lateral views. The child will be asked to take a deep breath so that the lungs are fully expanded. Some time before the X-ray is scheduled it is a good idea for parents to have the child practice taking a deep breath, holding it as the parents count to three, and then exhaling. Any child with a history of recurring or persistent chest symptoms including chronic cough, wheeze, shortness of breath, and persistent tightness of chest is a candidate for a chest X-ray.

- Sinus X-rays. May be ordered when there are recurring episodes of dizziness and pain located in the forehead and under the eyes, or for symptoms of chronic foul-smelling nasal discharge. In general, sinus X-rays will not be ordered for children less than 5 years of age, as these areas are not sufficiently developed in younger children. The radiologist will examine the X-rays for the presence of fluid within the sinuses, indicating improper drainage and the probability of infection; blockage of the sinus passages resulting from recurring infection; cysts or polyps growing in the sinus areas; thickening of the membranes lining the sinuses (a sign of either chronic infection or allergic stimulation).
- Side or lateral X-ray view of the neck. May be done as a check for chronically enlarged adenoids. Not ordered very often.
- Upper or lower intestinal tract X-rays. Used to evaluate the presence of chronic gastrointestinal complaints such as vomiting, nausea, diarrhea which might possibly have an allergic cause, i.e., from a food allergy. A barium containing contrast material is swallowed and films are then taken.

PURPOSE   To search for the cause of specific stomach or intestinal complaints.

HOW ADMINISTERED   By conventional X-ray equipment.

FREQUENCY   With chronic chest complaints an X-ray is frequently ordered. Sinus films are taken in older children and adolescents with persistent headaches. Gastrointestinal films are done infrequently, generally only with chronic or severe stomach or intestinal complaints.

PAIN   None.

COMMENTS   Though the safety of X-ray technology has been immensely improved through the years, it is still sound policy to ask the doctor what information she hopes to obtain from this test. Be very skeptical if the doctor's answer is too general or too vague. Any patient who enters the office with mild chest symptoms and some nasal symptoms should not be sent for X-rays immediately. If an X-ray study has been done recently, it may be unnecessary to repeat it.

Barium Swallow

PURPOSE   To find any unusual anatomical relationship existing between the feeding pathway (the esophagus) and the air passageway (the trachea); to find an improperly functioning junction at the point where the esophagus meets the stomach; to find an abnormal connection between the esophagus and the trachea, the result being the formation of an anatomical abnormality known as a tracheo-esophageal (T-E) fistula; if such a connection has formed, food may be backing up into the lungs, causing symptoms which cannot be readily distinguished from those of asthma. Gastro-esophageal reflux, another condition that can cause asthma symptoms, can be diagnosed with a barium swallow.

HOW ADMINISTERED   The child is asked to swallow a chalky barium mixture. The mixture is then X-rayed as it moves down the esophagus to the stomach similar to a standard X-ray except that many more exposures are made at a single session and the test may last for up to thirty minutes.

FREQUENCY   This test is ordered only when the doctor is suspicious that a fistula exists or the gastroesophageal junction is not functioning properly.

PAIN   No pain of any kind. The young child may, however, become restless or uncomfortable during the picture-taking session. The chocolate-flavored barium mixture is usually quite palatable to the child.

Magnification X-Rays of Upper Airways

PURPOSE   To examine with magnification the trachea and main branches of the bronchial tubes. The test is used to get an enlarged view of the anatomy of the major breathing passageways. This procedure can detect a variety of congenital structural abnormalities such as vascular rings, which can compress the esophagus and trachea.

FREQUENCY   Uncommon. Ordinarily this test is called for only when there is suspicion that a foreign object has been swallowed—coins, food, a blade of grass—and that this object has become lodged in the airways, producing asthmalike symptoms.

PAIN   None.

In Vitro Tests

The term *in vitro* literally means "in a glass" or "in a test tube"—figuratively, it describes a procedure that takes place in an environment *outside* the body. In vitro tests are therefore carried out in a laboratory rather than being performed directly on the patient.

RAST Test (Radioallergosorbent Test)

PURPOSE   An in vitro technique for measuring the circulating level of a specific IgE antibody (i.e., anti-ragweed IgE antibody) in the bloodstream. This test determines the level of potential sensitivity to a variety of specific allergens, including pollens, animals, molds, foods, and inhalants.

HOW ADMINISTERED   By venipuncture. The blood sample is divided into many small test tubes, each one containing a different antigen, i.e., tree pollen, ragweed pollen, dog dander, dust, wool, milk, etc. These specimens are then analyzed in a machine designed to detect either color changes in the tested substance or the degree of radioactivity in each tube. The procedure is performed using a system that detects changes in the color of a particular test sample or by means of radioactively tagged allergens.

PAIN   Mild momentary discomfort.

HOW COMMON   A frequently performed test.

COMMENTS   The appeal of RAST testing is that many tests can be performed from one blood specimen; a doctor can identify a wide spectrum of possible allergic sensitivities from analysis of a single laboratory sample, making it unnecessary for the child to return for further tests. The disadvantages of RAST testing are that the method is less sensitive than direct skin testing (see below) and a good deal more expensive.

PRIST Test (Paper Radioimmunosorbent Test)

PURPOSE   A general screening test to determine the patient's total IgE level. The RAST test determines individual levels of specific IgE antibodies; the PRIST test only determines the total amount of circulating IgE.

HOW ADMINISTERED   Venipuncture.

PAIN   Mild momentary discomfort.

HOW COMMON   The PRIST test is very commonly performed in the evaluation of a patient suspected of having an allergic problem. It is a good screening procedure. When a RAST test is done, a total IgE level is also obtained.

In Vivo or Direct Skin Tests

Skin tests performed directly on the patient are known as *in vivo* tests, i.e., tests carried out on a person rather than in the lab.

Epicutaneous Testing (Skin Tests)

PURPOSE   To determine allergic sensitivities to specific allergens.

HOW ADMINISTERED   By scratch, and prick technique.

The *scratch test* is done by making a row of superficial (and bloodless) scratches on the skin with a needle. A drop of a specific antigen extract —ragweed extract, dog extract, shellfish extract, etc.—is placed directly on one of the scratches and absorbed. A different antigen is then placed on the second scratch, another on the third, and so on. Each test site is numbered or otherwise labeled so that the antigen can be identified. Ten of these scratches may be made at one time on the forearm, or in some cases along the upper part of the back, usually in vertical rows. If the child has been sensitized to any of the specific allergens, a red, swollen hivelike bump will soon appear at that specific test site. The degree of reaction is then graded on a one-to-four scale: the larger, redder and more dramatic the bump, the greater the sensitivity. Twenty, or at most, thirty scratch tests may be done at a single testing session.

In the prick technique, a drop of antigen is placed on the forearm. The test site is then pricked with a needle, allowing the antigen to make contact with the tissue mast cells. A positive response consists of localized itching, swelling and redness on the test site. The patient who demonstrates such a reaction has been sensitized to the specific test substance placed on that spot. Ten to thirty prick tests can be done during an office visit. The usual test site is the forearm. Prick testing is a somewhat more sensitive method than scratch testing and is probably the best of all in vivo methods for food testing.

These tests are administered in the allergist's office. If reactions occur, they usually take place within ten to twenty minutes after the tests have been performed.

HOW COMMON A standard allergist's test. Both the scratch and the prick tests are first-line diagnostic allergy procedures, and they are effective techniques. When direct food testing is done, the prick test is the current method of choice.

PAIN The pain is no greater—and lasts no longer—than any other kind of scratch or pinprick. Most children take the momentary discomfort easily in stride. In the hands of a competent, concerned doctor, anxiety and pain response is minimal.

POTENTIAL DANGERS Although there are rarely problems related to this type of testing, the child is being tested for substances to which she may be allergic. This means that in addition to the local response on the arm —which feels and looks no worse than a large mosquito bite—the test material on rare occasions may trigger a more generalized allergic reaction. When this occurs, symptoms can take many forms: hives, general itching, sneezing, teary eyes, even asthma. Such a reaction is an extremely rare situation and responds dramatically to treatment given in the allergist's office.

COMMENTS The direct or in vivo skin test is one of the most sensitive and specific ways we have for detecting allergic sensitivities. A positive test indicates *only* that the patient has been *sensitized* to the test substance and therefore has the potential to develop allergic symptoms on reexposure to that allergen. Understand that this is *not* incontrovertible proof of a clinical allergic sensitivity. To come to this conclusion, the doctor must evaluate the entire history, physical condition and testing records of the child.

Intracutaneous or Intradermal Testing (literally, "within the layers of skin")

PURPOSE To determine specific allergic sensitivities to particular allergens.

HOW ADMINISTERED An antigen is injected into the superficial layers of the skin. Injections are applied approximately an inch apart in rows on the forearm or occasionally the upper back. If a reaction takes place, it will occur ten to twenty minutes after the injection.

HOW COMMON   A standard allergy testing procedure. Once performed it is usually not necessary to repeat this test. Only if there is a *significant* change in the child's symptoms should he be called in for further testing. I have never understood why some patients have been tested on a yearly basis when there has been no worsening of their symptoms or obvious change in the clinical course. I can think of no scientific reason to justify the constant retesting of patients who are progressing satisfactorily.

PAIN   Mild momentary discomfort. The pain associated with intradermal testing in the hands of a well-trained individual working with a cooperative patient usually causes minimal discomfort.

POTENTIAL DANGERS   In order to minimize the possibility of either a large local reaction or a more generalized response, the testing is started with highly diluted allergen mixtures. Nonetheless, the same small chance of a general allergic reaction that exists for epicutaneous testing (described above) also is present here.

COMMENTS   The intracutaneous technique is the most sensitive of all skin tests, *except* in the case of food allergies, where false responses to tested materials are common. If skin testing for foods is to be done at all, the best method to employ is the prick technique.

Patch Testing

PURPOSE   Used to evaluate substances suspected of causing allergic-type skin problems. It is particularly effective in identifying the metal and chemical allergies which cause contact dermatitis.

HOW ADMINISTERED   A piece of soft cloth or paper is impregnated with the suspected allergen. The patch is then applied directly to the skin of the patient's forearm or back and is covered with an adhesive bandage–type dressing. The test substance is left on for 48 hours and is then removed. A positive response consists of itching with redness and blistering of the skin at the test site.

FREQUENCY   Patch testing is sometimes done by the allergist; however, more commonly it is performed in a dermatologist's office. In general, an allergist may refer patients suffering from any unusual skin conditions to a dermatologist.

PAIN   Rarely. The usual response consists of localized itching and possible blister formation at the test site.

Oral Challenge Food Testing

PURPOSE   To confirm a suspected allergic sensitivity to a particular food substance.

HOW ADMINISTERED   Allergists do not yet have any totally accurate, easily performed testing methods for food allergies. The best system that exists is direct food challenge testing. This form of dietary manipulation calls for the removal of specific suspected foods or food groups from the child's diet: milk or oranges, for example. The patient is then observed to see if the allergic symptoms disappear. If symptoms do decrease, the patient is given the specific food again. If the symptoms reappear, this is good evidence of an allergic reaction. If the test is done twice with the same results, it is proof positive. In this case the expression "the proof of the pudding is in the eating" is an especially appropriate motto.

PAIN   If the test is positive, the patient can experience a variety of allergic symptoms.

HOW COMMON   A standard test.

POTENTIAL DANGERS   If the original reaction to the suspected food was very severe, with breathing problems, severe vomiting or diarrhea, then it is potentially quite dangerous to carry out a direct food challenge test. If it is absolutely essential to do this test, it must be carried out under direct medical supervision, preferably in a hospital setting. In this situation a challenge procedure is definitely *not* a medical do-it-yourself project.

Frequently Performed Tests

Pulmonary Function Study

PURPOSE   To judge how well the lungs are performing. Generally used by an allergist when dealing with asthmatic patients.

HOW ADMINISTERED   The child is asked to breathe into a mechanical device of some kind; there are many varieties. Like blood pressure readings, "normal" lung function values fall within a range which varies with a person's age, height, race and sex. A child who suffers from asthma will probably have some abnormal lung function values, even if there have been no recent symptoms.

PAIN   No pain.

HOW COMMON   Commonly performed with asthmatic children. The test may be done repeatedly, throughout the child's course of treatment. In serious cases it might be checked monthly. For a child who is progressing at a normal rate, pulmonary testing is done approximately every three to six months.

COMMENTS   A doctor may listen to a child's lungs through a stethoscope and find the patient's chest to be totally clear. This does not, however, indicate how well the child's lungs are actually functioning; a patient can have serious asthma and between attacks have totally clear-sounding lungs.

Sweat Test for Cystic Fibrosis

PURPOSE   Cystic fibrosis, or CF, is a genetically transmitted disease in which there is an abnormality in such glandular organs as the pancreas, salivary glands, sweat glands and mucus glands of the intestinal and respiratory systems. The symptoms, which include a cough, production of very thick mucus secretions and occasional wheezing, can under certain circumstances mimic those seen in asthma. For this reason the presence of cystic fibrosis must first of all be ruled out in young children before proceeding to make a diagnosis of asthma.

HOW ADMINISTERED   Children who are suffering from CF have exceedingly high levels of sodium chloride in their sweat. This imbalance can be detected by placing a piece of gauze on the child's arm and stimulating the sweat glands with a very low grade electrical current. The wrapping is left on the arm for about an hour and then removed. The sweat content is analyzed for the amount of sodium chloride it has produced.

HOW COMMON   This test is necessary only if a child has chronic respiratory symptoms similar to those found in cystic fibrosis.

PAIN   None.

After the Tests Are Completed

Once the appropriate tests have been completed, the findings are used in conjunction with the child's history and examination records to reach a final diagnostic conclusion, and to then formulate a plan of treatment. This treatment may involve one or all of three main therapeutic approaches. These are: environmental control; pharmacotherapy, the use of a wide range of medicines to control the child's allergic symptoms; immunotherapy, or allergy injection treatment to build up the child's resistance and immunity to specific allergen(s).

We will go into all three forms of allergy treatment in the next chapter. Remember: the presence of a positive reaction to any allergen during a test does not *necessarily* mean that a child is actually allergic to this substance. It does mean that the child has at some point in his life been exposed to this particular allergen, and sensitization to this substance has occurred. Once the child has been sensitized, then production of specific anti-dog IgE antibodies —or specific anti-ragweed IgE or whatever—provides him with the capability to develop allergic symptoms to these specific substances. Such a response can take place today, tomorrow, in ten years, or never. One simply never knows. Yet how common it is for a young patient to walk out of my office announcing that "I'm allergic to trees, grass, and feathers," when all that has really been established is that she has tested positively to these substances. Only after a doctor has evaluated *all* the clinical evidence can the child, the parents, and the doctor be sure that an allergy is really present.

How an Allergist Treats Your Allergic Child

Environmental Control

Whenever possible, the best way to stop allergic symptoms is to avoid the source of the problem. This approach is called environmental control. For example, if it has been determined that your child is allergic to dust or the pet dog, then elimination or avoidance of these allergens will be a big help in controlling your child's symptoms. This sounds simple and pat, and it is. Yet it's amazing how many parents overlook environmental control, even when a few easy changes might remedy a lifetime of allergic misery. The fact is that many allergic children can significantly decrease their symptoms merely by having suspected allergens removed from their living area; or, in certain cases, by removing the children themselves from the problem area. Whenever it can be practiced, preventive medicine is the best medicine.

For example, Richie, a thirteen-year-old boy, was recently brought to my office because for the first time in his life he was experiencing severe allergic symptoms: sneezing, tearing eyes and a maddening itch in the back of his throat. These symptoms had come on suddenly and with surprising violence a month and a half before his visit, and they were now continuing day after day without letup.

In the course of taking the boy's history I soon determined that one aspect of his life had changed: he had been given a long-haired collie about a month before his symptoms started. I did a skin test and found that the boy had a strong positive response to dog dander. I explained the situation to his family, and they all agreed to part with the dog on a trial basis. Within two weeks after the animal had left the home Richie's symptoms disappeared entirely.

Allergic symptoms do not always vanish with such ease, of course, and in many cases it is impossible to move away entirely from the source of an allergen. What cannot be avoided, however, usually—I say *usually*—can be manipulated, and this is the key to the practice of environmental control.

Dust, for example, is ubiquitous and a nemesis for millions of allergy-prone children. Contrary to popular notion, it is not composed of dirt or soil but a combination of the breakdown products of organic materials: animal dander, wool and linen fibers, feathers and plant residues. The dust in my house will be different from the dust in your house depending on how often you clean, whether you keep a pet, whether you raise plants, and so on.

One of the inhabitants of dust is an organism known as the dust mite, a quasi-microscopic insect that abides quite happily in the residences of rich and poor alike—it is no respecter of fine living. We all have an ample collection of these mites in our households, generally in the bedroom and specifically in our pillows, blankets and mattresses (the mites feed upon the tiny flakes of skin that fall from our bodies while we sleep). Disconcerting? Perhaps. But every home has its share of dust mites, and if kept policed they do no harm, except of course to those with dust allergies. For such people environmental control is imperative.

How can environmental control be carried out? In several ways.

Electronic Air Control Devices

Air conditioners are found in many homes today and are especially effective in the home of allergy sufferers, specifically for those children who have sensitivities to airborne allergens such as dust, mold spores or pollens. Not only do air conditioners partially filter out particles of dust and pollen but they cool the air and lower its humidity. Keep your air conditioner's surface free of molds and fungi by washing it frequently, changing the filter, and spraying it occasionally with a disinfectant. Unless the materials that get trapped in the filter are removed periodically, they can build up and leak back into the room. Also, be heedful of air conditioner machines that leak water, even small amounts. These droplets will add up and eventually become breeders of mold spores.

While air conditioners are helpful, they tend to filter out only larger particulate matter, such as mold spores and some pollens. Some of the more efficient machines have the capacity to remove airborne allergens in the 10- to 15-micron range. To give you some idea of the relative size of a micron, there are 25 millimeters in an inch and one micron is equal to 1/1000 of a millimeter. It's not very large! Special air filtering devices are required to remove airborne particles smaller than 5 microns (cigarette smoke, bacteria and metallic fumes). If you want complete protection from such irritants, you'll need an electronic air cleaner to supplement your air conditioner.

Electronic air cleaners come in many sizes and styles. One popular variety, the electrostatic unit, contains a built-in high voltage plate that continually exerts an electromagnetic charge on room air, drawing local dust particles into its filter in much the same way that a magnet attracts iron filings. The method, called electrostatic precipitation, is extremely effective, but the exhaust systems of some models emit ozone, an unstable gas potentially irritating to asthma sufferers. I know of several young asthmatics whose condition took a mysterious turn for the worse practically on the day that an electrostatic air cleaner was brought into their homes. The remedy was simply to exchange the ozone-producing model for one without this potentially annoying side effect. Even better relief is provided by air cleaners that work with the HEPA-type filter, a system developed by the space program for cleaning the atmosphere inside spacecraft. These machines produce no potentially irritating by-products, and, though expensive, clean the air with impressive efficiency.

Humidifiers, dehumidifiers and vaporizers. A *humidifier* is used in the winter when heating units dry out the air, robbing the atmosphere of essential water vapor. Too much of this artificial dryness will eventually cause the protective mucus barriers in the nose and throat to crack, thereby making the inhabitants of the household vulnerable to viral and bacterial infections. Schoolchildren who complain of sore throats every winter morning are not necessarily malingering; they may simply be having difficulty differentiating between what is infected and what is irritated. One way of beating "winter nose and throat" is to attach a humidifier directly to your heating unit. This unit will force water vapor *directly* into the atmosphere along with the heat and keep the indoor humidity at a comfortable level. If you do not have a forced-air heating unit, you can purchase a freestanding humidifier at any large appliance store and run it regularly during the cold, dry months. Look for a machine equipped with a *humidistat* which turns itself on and off automatically. The newest and most efficient room humidifier is the ultrasonic variety. The aerosol mist produced by this unit is so fine that it stays suspended in the air for long periods of time. Consequently, the room does not become cold and damp, a condition that occurs quite often with other types of room humidifiers. The ultrasonic units operate completely silently. This feature can be quite important for the child who has a problem falling asleep.

If it is not possible to purchase a humidifier, some improvement will be provided if shallow, relatively wide pans of water are placed close to the heating units.

Between 35 and 45 percent relative humidity is an ideal environment for human beings. Anything much above this and the atmosphere becomes predisposed to mold growth, especially undesirable in the home of any allergic child. High humidity may also aggravate asthma symptoms, which is why some asthmatics are more uncomfortable during hot, humid weather. In such instances a *dehumidifier* in the patient's room or in several strategic locations throughout the house and especially the basement is the best defense against dampness. A dehumidifier works by pulling water vapor out of the atmosphere, much in the manner of a mechanical sponge. Too much water in the air is just as debilitating as too little, and both extremes are potentially dangerous for allergic children. Dehumidifiers are especially useful in basements used as playrooms for youngsters. If there are damp areas upstairs, molds will tend to lurk here, too, and a dehumidifier will keep them at bay. During the sticky summer months a dehumidifier or an air conditioner can be placed in one room of the house to provide the allergy sufferer a haven against high humidity. Dehumidifiers cost between $100 and $250, depending on the extra bells and whistles they come with, such as automatic shutoff control or a built-in thermostat. They are expensive, but a worthwhile investment for any family with an allergic child.

The *vaporizer,* a device that emits a fine, steady spray of water vapor into the air, is useful in cases when sneezing, coughing and general allergic symptoms have dried out mucous membranes in the nose and head. There are two types of vaporizers, the cool mist and the steam. Generally speaking, steam vaporizers today have almost no place in the home of an allergic child. Their only real use is to treat a child with croup, and then a heated, steamed-up bathroom will do the job just as well. If you're using a vaporizer, the cool mist variety is unquestionably superior. In order to minimize the possibility that molds will grow in your humidifier unit, you must clean them thoroughly and regularly. One method is to run a dilute solution of Clorox and water through the unit and follow this with plain water. When you run the bleach solution through the machine, place it in a closed room with the window open so the bleach-containing water vapor will be vented outdoors. Repeat this procedure every one to two weeks.

Other suggestions for keeping the indoor air as inhalant free as possible include the following:

Place (and frequently replace) a new filter on your forced-air heating units.

Install filters on the outflow exits of the heating ducts in every room in the house. These filters can be homemade from several layers of cheesecloth; a regular furnace-style filter can also be used.

Install central air conditioning, keeping the filters well cleaned and maintained.

Manipulation of the External Environment

There are many modifications you can make in your child's surroundings, many of which are simple to do and most of which are surprisingly effective.

In certain cases a few modifications may be *all* that is necessary to control allergic symptoms.

Make a household room check. By carefully going through each room in your house or apartment you can remedy many conditions which can aggravate or trigger allergy symptoms. The living room, for instance, usually has more furniture in it than any other room. Keep all tables, chairs, bookcases, blinds, curtains, couches and bric-a-brac dust free, and vacuum the rugs at least twice a week. Watch out for wool-covered and overstuffed furniture, especially old furniture; both may be potential allergy hazards. You may wish to encase such furniture in protective coverings. In dens and offices, books are legendary collectors of dust if not gone over frequently with a rag or vacuum cleaner. Flocked wallpaper is also a potential allergic hazard because it attracts dust. Cooking odors from the kitchen may cause allergic symptoms; a good exhaust fan over the stove can remedy this problem. Bathroom tiles should be kept scrubbed and disinfected to eliminate mold, especially those located around the sink, tub and other damp spots. There are a number of effective sprays on the market that will kill molds before they become a problem. Your local supermarket or hardware store will be able to supply you with the names of these products. Basement areas may hold pockets of dampness that contribute to mold growth, which a dehumidifier will eliminate. Clothes dryers should be adequately vented to prevent dust and lint from recirculating through the house. Each house is different, of course, and has different logistic problems. Check each room, and make appropriate modifications when needed.

Choose rugs and furnishings wisely. If you're going to use carpeting in a child's room, make sure it is a low pile, nonwool, synthetic variety. The padding beneath the rug should be made of foam rather than a hair-type material. Furniture is less likely to cause allergic symptoms if it is stuffed with foam rubber rather than kapok or feathers. Replace heavy drapes with washable curtains. Avoid animal materials such as mohair, wool or horsehair.

Dustproof the child's bedroom. Approximately half of a young child's day is spent in her bedroom, so the necessity for dustproofing an allergic child's bedroom is self-evident. Get rid of all pillows and mattresses stuffed with kapok or down and replace them with foam- or polyester-stuffed varieties. Upholstered box springs should be avoided; they attract dust. The ideal sleeping arrangement for an allergic child is a platform-style bed or a bed with metal springs with all pillows and boxsprings enclosed in dustproof casings. Special dustproof mattress covers are helpful too, but shun headboards covered with fabric or upholstery. The child's blankets should be made of polyester or cotton. Be careful of the wool varieties—even if they do not promote allergies directly, they can be great dust catchers. Keep the door of the child's room closed when not occupied and try to vacuum the room at least every other day. Closed bookcases and closet doors that seal shut are helpful, as are washable curtains. Do not store toys or bric-a-brac under the bed or in any enclosed spot where dust accumulates, and remove damp clothes from the room, as well as mothballs, plants, perfumes, insect sprays, and hobby chemicals such as glue and paint. Dust mites, incidentally, cannot survive extremely low temperatures: If you live in a northern climate, airing a child's mattress and bed coverings on a sunny winter day will have an antiseptic effect as well as a freshening one. Vacuuming the mattress once a week will help reduce the dust mite population.

Maintain adequate temperature control. Avoid extremes of heat or cold. In the winter the indoor temperature should be maintained between 68 and 72 degrees Fahrenheit. In the summer, air conditioning is the best bet. Become weather-wise, and plan the child's activity schedule around the good days and the bad.

Clean your house often and with a special eye toward reducing dust. Clean all rooms thoroughly, especially those where the child spends much time. Always use the vacuum cleaner or a damp mop; avoid feather dusters or brooms. Disinfectants are all right for scrubbing, but first be sure the child is not allergic to them. Keep the child's room as uncluttered and airy as possible, and furnish it with substances posing no allergic danger: wood furniture; curtains of synthetic materials; plastic toys and furnishings; linoleum, wood, vinyl or tile floors; Formica desks and shelves; washable enamel paint on the walls, etc. Likewise, shun materials such as rattan, cane, velour, fur, wicker, mohair, wool, and so on, and be wary of stuffed animals. When vacuuming don't forget to concentrate on the dust-catching areas such as beneath the bed and across the venetian blinds. On major cleaning days it is wise to have the child leave the house for several hours because heavy cleaning raises the dust level temporarily.

Pets require special handling and consideration. Children with sensitivities to animals are obviously best off when the animals are removed from the house. For a variety of reasons, however, most of them psychological, the child and the animal may be inseparable. What you must do in this case is minimize contact. Vacuum the house frequently to remove animal hairs and shedding residues. The child's bedroom should be *absolutely, totally and always off-limits to the dog or cat,* and under *no* circumstances should the pet be allowed to sleep with the child or even climb up on his bed. The child must have an *absolutely animal-free sanctuary* in some section of the house for days when symptoms become intense, and if possible the animal should be housed outside much of the time.

Children are not allergic to animal hair or even to animal fur. What they are allergic to is the dander, the dead skin cells that constantly flake off the creature's body as the animal moves about. All animals produce dander, especially during the shedding season. Which means, despite the claims of some animal breeders, that there is no such thing as a nonallergenic dog or cat. To make matters worse, many children are allergic to the saliva of domestic animals, especially cats, and when licked by these animals severe allergy symptoms can occur. The salivary secretions from the family cat are deposited throughout the house. When the saliva dries, it becomes airborne and is inhaled by the allergic child, resulting in a continuing cycle of congestion, cough and possibly asthma. The most positive thing that can be said about the animal allergy situation is that certain breeds of dog or cat may affect some children more than others. Patterns of allergic response differ from child to child, and only a bit of careful sleuthing can establish which animals are likely to produce symptoms and which are not. Sensitivity to an animal does not necessarily mean that pets can never be admitted into the home. But certainly a good deal of guarded control will be necessary if they are.

Dietary Control

There is no such thing as a completely nonallergenic food; someplace, some-time, any food you can think of may cause an allergic reaction. Nevertheless, there are more common offenders.

They include:

nuts
dairy products: milk, cheese, cream, etc.
citrus fruits: oranges and grapefruit
cereal grains, primarily wheat
fruits, especially strawberries
sweets, especially chocolate
shellfish, especially shrimp and lobster
eggs

By removing a specific food suspected of causing an allergic reaction, you should be able to eliminate the source of the problem. See the chapter on food allergies (p. 167) for a full discussion.

Stinging Insect Control

The common stinging insects—the honeybee, the yellow jacket, the hornet, and the wasp—all belong to the biological order Hymenoptera of the class Insecta. Another nonwinged member of the group is the fire ant, which is the cause of growing concern primarily in the southeastern United States.

Again, avoidance is the key. Yellow jackets build nests in the ground, in tall grass, on lawns, or under stones. Hornets produce their familiar, gray, football-shaped wattle nests in tree branches or hang them from the eaves of roofs. Of all the allergy-producing insects, these are the most aggressive, tending to sting without provocation. Wasps are more docile and build smaller, honeycomb-type nests, also in trees and sidings. While the American honeybee is located mostly in artificial hives today, many natural nests can still be found in tree trunks and under the floorboards of older houses, barns or other enclosed areas.

Stings from these insects usually produce nothing more serious than a local reaction: a welt or a small swelling. This lesion does not constitute an allergic reaction but is a normal response to toxic substances contained in the insect venom. An allergic reaction occurs when a sting on one area—say, the leg—causes problems in other areas of the body, such as swelling on the arms or the face, hives across the torso, or difficulty in breathing. Severe reactions include significant breathing difficulties, a drop in blood pressure, unconsciousness, shock, and, on occasion, death. (There are approximately 50 to 75 reported deaths a year caused by allergic insect reactions resulting in anaphylaxis.)

Depending on the allergy, insect-sensitive children should:

Avoid contact with the nest. This of course includes steering clear of beehives, as well as any natural nook and cranny where bees build their hives: the tops of branches, hollow trees, stumps, etc.

Stay away from fields and orchards in flower; these are special haunts of nectar-seeking honeybees.

Avoid gardening. Yellow jackets frequently build nests in open, grassy areas. Anyone who has mowed over, dug up or unwittingly tripped over the underground homes of these nasty insects knows how ferociously they deal with intrusion. And staying outside for prolonged periods near flowering plants is inviting trouble from honeybees.

Steer clear of areas where organic wastes are stored. Yellow jackets and wasps regularly patrol dumps, refuse piles, garbage cans and compost heaps.

Don't stay outdoors where food is being kept or served. Stinging insects are frequently uninvited visitors to barbecues and picnics.

Don't use perfumes, cologne, scented hair tonics and scented deodorants. The odors from all these substances attract stinging insects. Avoid applying these or any other sweet-smelling potions to your child, especially if much time is being spent outdoors.

Don't dress in brightly colored clothing. Strong primary colors, the natural colors of flowers such as greens, yellows and reds, attract many stinging insects. It might be mentioned in passing that mosquitoes are especially fond of the color blue.

If your child has been diagnosed as being allergic to any of the Hymenoptera, keep an *insect sting kit* with you at all times. The older child should be instructed how to properly use the kit. The contents of the kit include antihistamine tablets and a pre-filled syringe containing epinephrine. It is especially useful for allergic children who are entering forested areas or who spend much time outdoors. An alternative to the sting kit is a product called the Epi-Pen, sold by Center Labs, a disposable, preloaded, pressure-activated syringe that automatically injects adrenaline when pressed against the skin. With a physician's prescription, sting kits and the Epi-Pen can be purchased at drugstores or from mail-order distributors. (See Appendix for addresses.)

Pharmacotherapy

The second of the three main treatment methods used by allergists, pharmacotherapy, involves the use of various oral, injected or inhaled medications. Almost every patient treated for an allergic condition will be given some type of symptomatic medication, and indeed, pharmacotherapy is by far the most frequently employed treatment method used for the control of allergic symptoms.

Five main categories of drugs are commonly used. At this point a review will help you identify their names and recognize their functions. Later, in the sections on individual allergic ailments, we will take a further look at each of these medicines from the standpoint of specific ailments: how they work, when their prescription is appropriate, what they can and cannot do for the allergic child, possible side effects, and so on down the list of essential considerations. Here are the five categories of drugs your child is likely to require.

Bronchodilators

These drugs relax the smooth muscle surrounding the bronchial tubes within the lungs. They are used almost exclusively for the treatment of bronchial asthma.

A number of individual drugs fall under this general heading. The most commonly used belong to a group called methylxanthines, and the most frequently prescribed of these is theophylline. Theophylline comes in a variety of forms, which are designated as short, intermediate and sustained action. It can be prescribed for children from infancy and can be used at any age. Other xanthine preparations include oxtriphylline (Choledyl), aminophylline and dyphylline. All these drugs except dyphylline are converted in the body to theophylline.

Another popular type of bronchodilator, the beta-adrenergic agents, includes prescription drugs such as metaproterenol, terbutaline and albuterol. The xanthines and the adrenergic agents work through different pharmacologic pathways, but both ultimately bring relief to asthma sufferers in the same way, by relaxing and dilating the breathing tubes when they are in spasm.

A third class of bronchodilator drugs, the anticholinergic agents, are being actively investigated and will gradually become available for general use. Representative examples of this class of drugs are atropine sulfate and iprotropium bromide (Atrovent). Currently these medications are only available in an aerosol form. For children, they are not the first line of antiasthma drugs.

Cromolyn Sodium

This drug is marketed in a variety of forms. The newest is the Intal inhaler, a metered-dose aerosol spray; it also comes in a capsule form that is inhaled from a device called the Spinhaler. These preparations are used to treat asthma. Nasalcrom, a pump-activated nasal spray, is used for allergic rhinitis. Finally, there is an ophthalmic form called Opticrom, which is useful for treating allergic conjunctivitis.

Cromolyn sodium are unique among antiallergy medicines in that their action is prophylactic: they have the ability to block allergic reactions *before* they begin. This means the drugs are helpful only as a preventive measure. If a person is having active symptoms, cromolyn sodium will generally be ineffective in providing relief.

Antihistamines

The most familiar of the antiallergy drugs, antihistamines act to inhibit the action of the chemical substance histamine and are mainly prescribed for the control of perennial and seasonal allergic rhinitis (hay fever). The term antihistamine does not, however, refer to a single drug or even to a particular class of drugs. In actuality there are six different classes of drugs, all of which fall under the antihistamine umbrella.

While most allergic individuals have taken an antihistamine at one time or another, some of the drug's subtle characteristics are not always understood. If, for instance, a certain class of antihistamine does not control your child's symptoms, don't give up, just try another from a different chemical group. This is an especially important point. Somewhere along the line the right preparation will be found, though quite often a trial-and-error approach must be taken before the most effective one is discovered.

Also worth remembering is that if a patient takes an antihistamine from group A and after a month or so the drug loses its effectiveness, a switch to group B antihistamines will often give continued relief. Then, after an appropriate amount of time has elapsed, the patient can return to the original antihistamine from group A and it will once again be effective.

Decongestants

These drugs help to shrink the swollen mucous membranes of the nose, especially in patients who are suffering from hay fever or animal dander allergies. Unlike many of the antihistamines, decongestants do not cause sleep-producing side effects nor will they interfere with the beneficial effects of antihistamines.

A word of warning is in order here concerning over-the-counter nasally administered decongestants: do not take these drugs for more than three to five days at a time. Continued use can lead to the worsening of the very nasal congestion you are trying to control; prolonged use may actually cause irreversible damage to the mucous membranes of the nose. There are more details on this in the section on hay fever (see page 146).

Corticosteroids

Cortisone is the best-known example of this potent group of anti-allergic drugs. It is a naturally occurring hormone produced normally by the adrenal glands in response to stress. Extremely useful in treating almost all types of allergic conditions ranging from asthma to itchy rash to chronic nasal problems, cortisone derivatives are available in a variety of forms—creams, ointments, tablets, aerosol sprays, nasal sprays, syrups and injectable solutions. Except for the weakest-strength creams, the corticosteroid drugs cannot be purchased over the counter and must be prescribed by a physician. Of all allergy drugs these are perhaps the most powerful *and* the most potentially dangerous. For more concerning their use, see the chapters on asthma, rhinitis, and allergic skin conditions.

Expectorants

Many allergic patients suffer from a chronic cough that produces a thick, sticky mucus that is difficult to cough up and spit out. Expectorant drugs, at least in theory, work on these secretions, helping to keep them in a more fluid state and allowing the patient to expel them with greater ease. Expectorants can be purchased over the counter at any drugstore, though in my opinion, fluids of any kind—especially plain water, hot or cold—are as good as most of the commercial preparations available today.

Physiotherapy and Exercise

Physical therapy is an important adjunct to the overall care of allergic children in general and asthmatic children in particular. Techniques can take the form of a specific set of breathing exercises taught to the child by a respiratory therapist, or they may involve a more general plan of participation in games and athletics.

As a rule, all allergic and especially asthmatic children should be encouraged to participate in physical activities appropriate to their age group and physical condition. Preventing a child with an allergic problem from becoming involved in normal play creates both a bad self-image and unavoidable conflict with other children. There are few more pathetic sights than that of a schoolchild sitting sullenly on the playground bench, passively watching friends romp during recess or in gym. Such a child quickly turns into the class outcast or invalid, and other children are rarely shy about rubbing it in.

Of course, physical activity in some children may cause the very symptoms you are trying to avoid, but there are almost always medications which keep these symptoms under control and which allow the child to play as children must. Activities which demand constant running such as soccer or basketball are more likely than others to trigger wheezing attacks, and the severely asthmatic child should probably steer clear of them. Other sports such as swimming, tennis, baseball and cycling are in general quite well tolerated and in many cases have a therapeutic effect on the child. Encourage them.

Finally, for children who suffer from bronchial asthma an adjunct therapy frequently recommended is an exercise called diaphragmatic breathing. This interesting technique teaches the child to use his diaphragm in such a way that deeper, more relaxed and effective breaths are taken, which helps to raise mucus secretions more easily from the lower parts of the bronchial tubes. I provide a specific exercise for diaphragmatic breathing (Belly Breathing) in the Appendix. Essentially, breathing exercises provide a relaxing diversion for the child with asthma. They will enable the youngster to better control asthma symptoms during an attack.

Immunotherapy

The last form of allergy therapy, referred to in the vernacular as "allergy shots," is technically known as immunotherapy and is the treatment people most often associate with the allergist's office. Immunotherapy consists of a program in which the child is given injections of the *particular allergens to which he is allergic.* Treatment is started with very low doses of these allergens; if the injections are well tolerated the dose is then increased in a controlled fashion up to a maintenance dose level. Children usually receive shots on a weekly basis for a period of from four to eight months. They then shift to an every-other-week schedule for approximately six months, then into an every-three-week schedule and so on to the point where injections are given once a month. Treatment is continued until a child is free of symptoms for approximately fifteen to eighteen months. At this point the treatment is considered to be successful and may be discontinued. The average course of treatment lasts for three to five years. If patients have been carefully selected, treatment results are generally quite good.

This state of decreased allergic reactivity (or responsiveness) is less permanent than the immunity developed for diseases such as smallpox and polio, and if symptoms recur immunotherapy must be repeated. The decision to start immunotherapy is made only after a careful evaluation of the patient if everyone is satisfied that neither environmental measures nor pharmacotherapy are adequately controlling the symptoms. The major conditions treated by immunotherapy include allergic seasonal and perennial rhinitis and, in certain cases, asthma. The number of allergy-causing substances one can be successfully immunized against is limited and specific. The list includes tree pollens, grass pollens, ragweed, dust, a variety of mold substances and in some cases animal dander. Sensitivities to allergens such as wool, feathers and especially foods should not be treated with immunotherapy.

Treating the Treated Child

In any situation where a child has chronic or recurring symptoms and is receiving special treatment, parental support and constant encouragement play a very important role in the overall management approach. Fortunately, most allergic conditions are not very severe and are more of an annoyance, a significant one at times, than a major problem. Still, such support is a significant part of the therapy itself.

The best steps parents can take after making sure their child is treated by a competent physician and ensuring that the household environment is friendly to allergy-free living is to be appropriately concerned when an attack occurs, to empathize as fully as possible with the child's psychological situation, and, above all, to remember what sickness of any kind was like for oneself as a child. Parents must also steer a narrow course between, on the one hand, overcoddling children when trouble starts and, on the other, becoming gradually callous and unresponsive to their complaints. Perhaps the most important of all virtues we can practice when dealing with an allergic child is sympathy tempered by common sense.

In some instances, of course, the situation is more demanding, as with severe asthma or eczema. In such cases there is almost certain to be dramatic impact on the life of the entire family. Depending on the age and temperament of the child, the handling of this situation must be different in different cases. No matter what approach is taken, however, it is of the greatest importance that the child be made to understand that he can and *must* lead as nearly normal a life as possible.

This means that overprotecting children or continually reminding them how sick they are is an urge to avoid. If you are going to err, do so on the side of permissiveness in matters such as participation in sports or vigorous activities, in allowing the child to hike, fish, camp and run free like other children. One of the more serious mistakes parents can make is to act as though their child were different—handicapped, crippled or odd—incapable of doing the things that other children do. The more a youngster is urged to participate in usual childhood activities, the less likely she will consider herself to be abnormal or different. The importance of providing a seriously allergic child with a strong, positive self-image cannot be overstressed.

Questions and Answers about Allergies and Allergists

How can I tell if an allergist is competent?

An allergist should have completed at least a two-year program of specialized training at an accredited allergy training center. Check to see that the doctor is certified by the American Board of Allergy and Immunology; this is one relatively easy way to know that he has passed intensive examinations and is well qualified. A recommendation from your pediatrician will usually lead you to a competent specialist. Most allergists who are members of the staff at a medical school or teaching hospital are highly competent physicians.

What is the best way to handle a child who is afraid of visiting an allergist?

As usual, honesty is the best policy with children. If your child is particularly uneasy about the upcoming visit, it is your responsibility to gather as much information as possible beforehand. This may require a phone call to the consultant's office, either to speak to the doctor's secretary-receptionist or even to the doctor concerning what will take place at the visit. This information should then be passed on to your child simply and directly. If your child continues to fear the visit, inform the doctor about it ahead of time to allow planning the examination and testing procedures accordingly.

What are some of the specific things you can tell children to relieve them of fear?

Probably the thing children fear most about a visit to the allergist's office is getting a "shot." Since the time injections first became a standard part of medical procedure, stories have circulated among children about needles at the doctor's office, some of which, no doubt, measure a foot long or maybe even two! Just the word "shot" itself conjures up images of guns and impact and pain.

From my experience the only way to remove a child's anxiety on this subject is to have the doctor carefully explain ahead of time exactly what he is and is not going to do. The doctor must approach this task in a relaxed, unhurried and sympathetic manner. Quite often I will do the first test on the parent so that the child can be an observer before becoming a participant.

In many cases the expectations of parents can be so great concerning a visit to the allergist that they unwittingly convey either a sense of anxiety to the child or an unrealistic anticipation of a "total cure." Neither is desirable. Simply tell the child that he will soon be visiting a doctor who has a particular interest in his allergy problem and who wants to find out what causes it, and to help it. Respond to all questions with simple, clear answers. Never evade a question, but don't get too technical, either. Be honest: if you know that a test is going to be done, and that it involves a particular procedure, say so.

The fact is that some children who visit an allergist have had previous exposure to allergy testing. If parents learn about these tests before coming to the office, if they discuss them with their child with assurance and honesty, if the doctor is not rushed or abrupt when administering them, and if time is taken at the initial visit to establish the all-important doctor-parent-patient relationship, the whole evaluation will prove to be a positive experience.

What is the best way to prepare a child for a long-term, ongoing series of treatments?

The tests and treatments at an allergist's office are usually neither frightening nor painful. I find that when children must be given weekly injections, most of them get used to the routine quickly, especially when they see for themselves what it actually entails. A child who kicks and screams whenever injection time rolls around is, in my experience, extremely rare. In fact, many children come to pride themselves on the brave, nonchalant manner they show when facing a needle.

Let me also say that the decision to prescribe long-term therapy will not come for at least several weeks after the initial consultation visit. If allergy injections (immunotherapy) are recommended, there is time over the course of these visits for the doctor to speak with the child, to establish a relationship, and for the parents to accustom the child to the notion of such treatment.

Is it wise for a doctor to talk about a child's condition in front of the child?

I feel a child should be involved in all discussions regarding her allergic condition. There are only very rare exceptions to this policy. Education of the entire family is one of the major contributions the physician can provide, and the more everyone knows about the specific problem the better the outcome will be for the patient. Children can assume much more responsibility for their own medical management than they have been given credit for.

How long will the first visit usually take?

This varies from doctor to doctor. An average consultation probably runs about an hour.

How expensive will it be?

Allergist's fees vary widely from doctor to doctor, from city to city, from state to state. They are by no means standardized. Consequently, it is difficult to quote a specific dollar amount for a consultation, especially since we are dealing with a wide spectrum of possible problems and treatments. "There are doctors and then there are doctors," as the saying goes. As a caveat to this bit of wisdom, however, remember also that the most expensive physician is not necessarily the best physician.

How then can the prospective patient determine what an allergist's fee will be? Simple: ask in advance. The parent should in fact gather as much information as possible concerning fees and ongoing medical expenses when first making the appointment. Forewarned is forearmed.

What if a doctor's office refuses to quote fees over the phone?

You then have a perfectly understandable reason for bypassing the doctor and going to the next. Most medical offices, however, will be happy to quote their fees ahead of time.

Can allergic symptoms change? For example, can an allergic skin condition become a nasal problem? Or a chest problem?

In some cases, yes. The development of allergic symptomatology is sometimes progressive. For example, quite often a young child will develop an allergic skin condition that disappears within twelve to twenty-four months. Once the skin problem vanishes, however, symptoms of allergic rhinitis or asthma may replace it. (This relationship between allergic skin conditions and nasal or chest symptoms has been called the dermal-respiratory syndrome.) There is no set pattern to the way these symptoms shift.

If allergic symptoms are neglected, will they worsen?

If symptoms are caused by exposure to a specific allergen and the child is constantly exposed to this substance without being treated, the child's symptoms will probably become more serious.

But there are other considerations to think about, too. If a child has an itchy rash and the parents do nothing to control it, the itching sensation will almost certainly worsen. Because of persistent scratching by the child the rash will spread and there is a good chance that it will become secondarily infected. Common sense would suggest that an ounce of prevention provided by early medical treatment will be worth more than a pound of cure afterward.

In the same regard, if a child suffers from allergic nasal symptoms and nothing is done to control them, the ailment will not necessarily become worse. But it *will* persist and it *will* become chronic and it *will* invite all the secondary woes such a chronic condition can bring: permanently chapped upper lip, red nose, itchy eyes, the exhaustion of incessant sneezing, and so on. Again, preventive medicine is the wisest course. Early medical treatment is clearly the best way—and really the only way—to treat an allergic symptom.

Certain allergic ailments—asthma in particular—unequivocally call for medical treatment right away, now, immediately and without delay. To assume that labored breathing is not a serious enough reason to warrant a trip to the doctor, or that the problem will go away on its own when the child gets older, is to look for trouble. What's more, one should not assume that after an asthmatic attack is over the child will never have a recurrence. Once the first asthma attack occurs, there is a good chance that other episodes will develop.

In essence then, parents are well advised to do *something* about allergic symptoms, even if it is only utilizing over-the-counter medications to achieve temporary relief. In most cases symptoms will get progressively worse without treatment. At best they will stay the same; and this is no pleasure for the child.

Are there any cases where medication is not necessary?

Leslie is five years old. She lives across the street from a friendly older widow who owns three friendly old cats. Whenever Leslie visits the woman and her pets—or when she visits anyone else who happens to own cats—the dander from the animals makes her sneeze.

Several hours after leaving the woman's house Leslie's symptoms vanish and they don't start up again until her next visit. Leslie's allergic reaction is relatively mild, and the pleasure she derives from playing with the animals, in her parents' estimation (and also, by the way, in her own), outweighs the temporary discomfort the contact brings. In such a case, when the allergen is native to a particular place and can normally be avoided, when the symptoms disappear quickly, and when the symptoms themselves are minor, then medication is not necessary.

Do children outgrow allergies?

Sometimes. While we are not certain what the term "outgrow" really means, we do know that over a period of time many children show a decrease in allergic symptoms, both in frequency and intensity. This does *not* hold true for everybody, specifically in the case of asthma. If we take a hundred five-year-old asthmatic children and observe them for a ten-year period, we will see that approximately a third of these children have no obvious asthma symptoms at ages ten to fifteen, that a third have remained the same, and that a third have gotten worse. Can we identify which child will fall into which of these categories? No. It's impossible for a doctor to look at a five-year-old and say, "You're going to get better" or "You're going to get worse."

At the same time some facts can assist the doctor in making what amounts to an educated guess. Family history of asthma, the course of the asthma condition since its start, and the patient's response to medication can sometimes suggest what direction the child's condition will take.

So one should never assume that with the passage of time children will automatically shed their allergies?

The chances are roughly one in three that they will. The situation can be an illusive one, too, as allergies sometimes go into a kind of remission during adolescence, only to reappear years later. Again, this is particularly true in the case of asthma. Bear in mind that there is nothing magical about the period of puberty which parents of allergic children await with such great anticipation. While many physical and hormonal changes do occur at this time, nature by no means guarantees that a reduction of allergic response will be one of them. Some children get better; some get worse. It's one of nature's many unfathomable lotteries.

Some parents assume that their child has outgrown a serious hay fever or bothersome skin condition when in fact she has simply been removed from its cause. If a child lives in the mountains, then moves to the city and the next year ceases to have attacks, this does not necessarily constitute a cure. To be fully sure that the child has "outgrown" a sensitivity, the child must return to the source of the allergen and continue to remain symptom-free.

Will childhood allergies ever disappear spontaneously, on their own?

Occasionally, but only occasionally, so don't bank on it. Better to work from the premise that the allergy will *not* disappear on its own; and then, if it happens to do so, give thanks that your child is among the fortunate few.

Are childhood allergies more common in one sex than in the other?

In early childhood, boys develop allergic symptoms more frequently than girls. During adolescence the graph reverses, and females statistically become more vulnerable. No one knows exactly why.

Can an allergic condition severely cripple or disable a child?

One day a five-year-old girl came into my office with a case of eczema so advanced that she was hardly able to walk. The creases behind her knees had become badly infected and it was almost impossible for her to bend her legs; she had to be carried into the examining room.

So the answer is yes, a child can be severely handicapped by an allergic disease, and this does not just include the most obvious instance of respiratory crippling that takes place in untreated asthma. Severe sneezing and tearing of the eyes during the hay fever season can, for instance, become so debilitating that the child ceases to function normally and may not be able to attend school. Most cases of this kind, it should be added, develop in children who have *not* been cared for by a physician in the early stages.

What is the most severe form of allergic reaction a child can develop?

It is known as anaphylaxis, a generalized reaction involving the skin, respiratory and cardiovascular systems of the body. An allergic child can develop anaphylaxis from exposure to any allergen to which he is sensitive. Symptoms consist of any one or all of the following: a generalized itchy rash (urticaria or hives), shortness of breath, tightness of the chest, wheezing (asthma), drop in blood pressure (hypotension) and loss of consciousness (syncope). Anaphylaxis is frequently associated with allergic reactions to foods, drugs, and insect stings. A true medical emergency, it calls for the *immediate* attention of a physician. If untreated, the outcome may ultimately prove to be fatal. With prompt medical treatment an anaphylactic reaction can be successfully controlled.

Under what circumstances can an allergic condition be fatal?

In certain rare cases. An anaphylactic reaction, as I've said, if untreated, has the potential to end in death. Also, a severe asthma attack has the capability of clogging the breathing passages with thick mucus plugs and suffocating the patient. It is estimated that around 3,500 people a year die from asthma, approximately 75 to 100 of them children. Between 50 and 100 people a year die from allergic reactions to insect stings.

Can a child who has not been treated for an allergy in its early stages recover sufficiently in the hands of a competent allergist if treated at a later date?

As a rule, the proper identification and avoidance of specific allergic sub-stances, along with the use of appropriate medications, can transform most children from passive observers of life into active participants. A new patient of mine was prevented from participating in her favorite sports because of a severe asthmatic condition. After being started on a proper management pro-gram with an appropriate bronchodilator drug, she quickly took up athletics again and eventually became the star of her volleyball team. The moral of this story and many others like it is that even the most severely asthmatic child can be significantly helped.

Will a rundown or sickly child be more likely to develop allergies than a healthy one?

There is at present no medical evidence to indicate that a debilitated child runs an increased risk of developing allergic symptoms. The causes of allergy seem to lie almost exclusively in genetic, cellular and environmental origins.

Is there an average age at which allergies begin to develop in children?

While the age of onset generally spans the spectrum of the childhood years, there is a tendency for certain conditions, specifically eczema and food aller-gies, to occur during the first years or even the first months of life. Problems such as hay fever tend to begin after the child is three or four. Asthma can develop at any time, from infancy to adolescence. Sensitivities to substances such as antibiotics, aspirin, insect stings and environmental pollutants can develop at almost any age.

Can a newborn child be allergic?

While it is theoretically possible for a newborn to become sensitized in utero and therefore respond allergically, such cases are quite unusual, indeed. I can, however, recall having seen a three-day-old infant develop allergic nasal congestion from drinking a milk-based formula. Other infants not infrequently develop intestinal symptoms such as diarrhea and vomiting after being fed a milk-based formula. I have also seen very young children develop eczema because of a food allergy.

How long does it usually take for an allergic reaction to appear once a child has made contact with an allergen?

It depends on the child's degree of sensitivity. In some situations the reactions will begin almost immediately after contact, particularly if the young person happens to be highly susceptible. Allergic symptoms can develop very rapidly or can evolve gradually over a period of hours following exposure to a specific allergen.

Are allergies ever contagious?

No, never. Allergic children sometimes develop a nasty-sounding cough mistakenly labeled bronchitis. The youngster is then sent home or kept out of school for no reason other than misdiagnosis. As a physician I am constantly writing notes to teachers, explaining that even though Johnny is sneezing his head off or coughing violently the problem is an allergic one, not an infectious one, and that it poses no threat to other children.

Part Two

The Treatment of Specific Allergic Conditions

Asthma

First the bad news: While we can't give exact numbers, it is estimated that between 9 and 10 million people in the United States today suffer from some form of bronchial asthma. Of this group, approximately 3,500 will die each year directly from the disease. Fortunately, the number of asthma fatalities occurring in children represents only a very, very small percentage of this figure! Another group, no one knows how large, will suffer from ailments to which it is a contributing cause. Among children, millions of school days will be lost each year because of asthma, and in many pediatric hospitals it will be one of the two or three most common ailments for which children are admitted. Indeed, concern for an asthmatic child will sometimes become so total that it dominates all aspects of family life, from vacation planning to the daily menu; every decision must eventually hinge on the inevitable question of whether it will conflict with Susie's "condition." So do not be fooled: asthma can be a serious matter. The cost in terms of time and money, disruption of family life and plain human suffering is impossible to calculate. It is not a condition to be minimized and certainly not one to be ignored.

On the other hand—and here's the good news—despite the many potential problems, the overwhelming majority of children with asthma can function normally. Their symptoms can be so well controlled that they will live active, healthy lives.

While asthma has been recognized as a medical condition since the time of Hippocrates, it is still difficult to come up with a definition that is accepted by all physicians. The ailment seems to be triggered by so many diverse agents, the symptoms can differ so widely among sufferers, and the actual cause of the sickness is still not completely understood that a definition on which everyone agrees continues to elude us.

Such lack of unanimity notwithstanding, the following simple definition covers most of the important aspects of this disorder and will serve adequately for our purposes.

Asthma is a reversible, obstructive airways disease.

Let's take a close look at this sentence.

Asthma is reversible. This means that almost always the severe breathing difficulties that occur during an asthma attack can, with proper treatment, be reversed to normal breathing patterns, and that permanent lung damage does not result from such attacks, even in the worst cases.

These are comforting facts for parents to recognize, that *the symptoms of asthma are not permanent,* and that *with proper treatment* they can *be reversed to a normal condition.* A diagnosis of asthma is by no means a sentence of doom or banishment from childhood fun. Today there are many professional and Olympic-class athletes who suffered with bronchial asthma as children, many opera singers, many ballet dancers, marathon runners and heavy-duty laborers, all of whom live normal lives today, their asthma kept well controlled by effective and appropriate medication.

Asthma is an obstructive condition. A child wheezes because the air passageways (bronchial tubes) are obstructed and therefore air cannot be easily expelled from the lungs. This obstruction is caused by three factors:

When an attack begins, the smooth muscles surrounding the breathing tubes (bronchi) go into spasm and tighten, thereby narrowing the bronchi.

When stimulated during an attack, the mucus glands lining the breathing passageways produce large amounts of very thick, sticky mucus (normal mucus is thin and watery in consistency). These increased secretions can block the smallest air passageways (respiratory bronchioles) and worsen the asthma attack.

Finally, because of inflammation and irritation within the smallest breathing passageways several things occur: there is swelling of the cells lining the bronchioles (the smallest bronchi) and a buildup of cellular debris from dead tissue cells, viruses and bacteria. The end result is a significant decrease in the size of the bronchial airways.

These three interdependent processes produce a wide range of physical symptoms. These include:

- tightness in the chest
- shortness of breath
- fatigue
- coughing
- wheezing
- anxiety
- most conspicuously, an inability to catch one's breath

It should be added that not every patient has all these symptoms during every attack. Still, everyone who experiences a mild asthma attack is aware that something decidedly unpleasant is taking place and that the lungs are by no means functioning as they should.

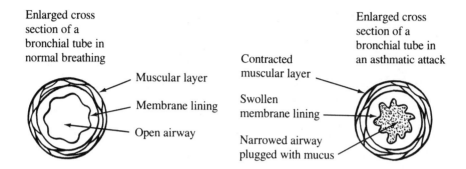

Enlarged cross section of a bronchial tube in normal breathing

Muscular layer

Membrane lining

Open airway

Contracted muscular layer

Swollen membrane lining

Narrowed airway plugged with mucus

Enlarged cross section of a bronchial tube in an asthmatic attack

The anatomy of asthma
SOURCE: National Heart, Lung, and Blood Institute

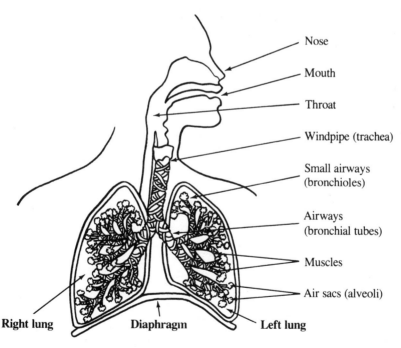

Nose

Mouth

Throat

Windpipe (trachea)

Small airways (bronchioles)

Airways (bronchial tubes)

Muscles

Air sacs (alveoli)

Right lung   **Diaphragm**   **Left lung**

Normal lungs

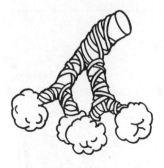 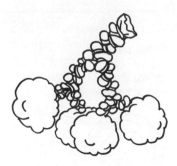

Inside the lungs during an asthma attack

CREDIT: National Heart, Lung, & Blood Institute

SOURCE: C.H. Feldman and N.M. Clark, *Open Airways/Respiro Abierto: Asthma Self-Management Program*, National Heart, Lung, and Blood Institute, NIH Publication No. 84-2365.

Asthma is a disease of the airways. It is in the bronchial tubes that the asthmatic process takes place. The disease is *not* centered in the air sacs whose job it is to take oxygen to the body and transport carbon dioxide for removal from the body. Asthma is strictly a disease of the breathing passageways.

Note that the word *allergy* does not appear in our definition, and for good reason: a child need not suffer from allergies to have asthma. His asthma may be triggered by either allergic or nonallergic causes.

Nonallergic asthma. Originally termed "intrinsic asthma" because there were no obvious external causes for the asthma. It was believed that the reason for the attack came from something *within* the person. Today it is recognized that there are many nonallergic triggers for asthma. A partial list includes: viral respiratory infections, changing weather patterns, strenuous physical exertion (especially in cold weather), stressful emotional situations, irritating odors and air pollution.

Allergic asthma. Allergic, or "external," asthma is triggered by allergens originating outside the body. It is caused by the typical allergens we have met so far—dust, pollen, dander, etc. To complicate the issue further, many patients have the ability to react asthmatically to both types of stimuli, the allergic and the nonallergic. Such children are diagnosed as having a "mixed" form of asthma. Asthma symptoms are the same regardless of the specific cause of an attack. Only after a complete allergy evaluation has been completed will it be possible to make a specific diagnosis regarding the cause(s) of your child's asthma.

The Symptoms of Asthma: What to Look For and What to Ignore

The perennial question, "Why does my child have asthma?" is still partially unanswerable. We do know that both genetic and environmental factors play a role, and that children with asthma have "hyperreactive airways" (some refer to them as "twitchy lungs"). Such supersensitive bronchial passageways are especially responsive to a variety of stimuli including allergens (dust, foods, pollens, animal danders, etc.), physical exertion, viral infections and emotional stress. Exposure to any of these triggers can rapidly bring on an asthma attack.

Bronchial hyperreactivity is thus the one physiological abnormality common to everyone with asthma. The situations or events that trigger asthma symptoms can vary greatly from one child to the next. For example, for some youngsters symptoms will be mostly associated with upper respiratory tract infections. Every time the child has a mild cold, an asthma attack will develop. Others show a clear pattern of asthma only at specific times of year. These children sometimes develop asthma secondary to reactions to mold spores or to specific pollens which are airborne during certain months, especially in the spring and fall. For yet another group of children, foods may be the triggering mechanism. For still others animal dander or feathers are the culprits.

Other causes of asthma? Take your pick: strenuous physical exercise; dampness or cold; cigarette smoke; extremely dusty environments; irritating odors; excessive laughter; strong winds; household chemicals; air pollution— the list goes on. For some patients only a few of these agents will cause problems. For others a panoply of potential asthma triggers lurk both in nature and around the house. And for a small minority of unfortunate individuals all the situations mentioned above, as well as others yet unlisted, can catapult these persons into a full-blown asthmatic attack.

Merely labeling a child as asthmatic doesn't say very much. As a physician I have seen children who wheeze only rarely, who have no trouble breathing, and who in fact show no other respiratory symptoms. Yet, clinically speaking, these children have bronchial asthma. At the other end of the spectrum, I have cared for children who in spite of all the effective antiasthma medicines available continue to wheeze and struggle for breath every day of their lives.

There is no single clinical pattern for the young patient with asthma. I constantly find myself telling parents of asthmatic children that the one consistent thing about asthma is its inconsistency. If you are the parent of an asthmatic child, it is important to keep this point in mind, that the pattern of asthma symptoms in this child and the pattern of symptoms in that child will not necessarily—and probably won't—be the same as the pattern of symptoms in *your* child.

Having said all this, here is a list of the possible symptoms that alone or together should heighten suspicion that your child may have asthma:

- wheezing, noted primarily when breathing out (expiration)
- complaints of tightness in the chest
- an inability to take a deep breath

- an inability to breathe comfortably while lying down
- complaints of chest and stomach pains
- a constant harsh cough

If any combination of these symptoms continue for more than twelve to twenty-four hours, consult your child's doctor. If you have no regular physician, a visit to a medical facility, either a hospital emergency room or a clinic, is your next step. At any time you feel your child's symptoms are obviously worsening, get some medical assistance either by telephone or a visit to the office.

There are additional points to bear in mind about identifying asthma symptomatology. Between attacks there are usually no abnormal physical findings when a child is examined by a physician. The symptoms of asthma can stay unusually well hidden until the hour of attack. It will often take special tests and equipment to detect respiratory abnormalities of any kind during symptom-free times.

Andy, aged ten, wheezes once or twice a year. Chris, who is eleven, has shortness of breath and a sensation of chest tightness several times a week. Here are two patients with bronchial asthma, and neither considers himself to be "sick." In Andy's case the conclusion is understandable. Chris's reaction is more surprising, perhaps, but it is also refreshingly healthy. The point is that most children with chronic asthma symptoms will wish to ignore their symptoms and get on with their lives. When such an attitude begins to emerge, parents are well advised to cooperate fully. In all but the most severe cases, asthmatic children should be encouraged to participate in a full range of social and athletic activities, and parents of these children should under no circumstances hold them back with ominous warnings about "strain" or "overdoing." In fact, it is an axiom: the less the asthma bothers the child, the less it should bother the parent.

If a child is old enough to have pulmonary function (breathing) studies done, most patients will show *some* detectable abnormalities of lung function. Even when the child displays no manifest symptoms, pulmonary function test abnormalities can show up. This is true even many years after a person has had his last attack. The true significance of this finding is not understood. An abnormal pulmonary function study may possibly indicate a poor prognosis later on in life. The final answer on this question is still up in the air.

During an attack, wheezing, noted mainly though not exclusively when exhaling, is *the* most common symptom of asthma and is by and large the hallmark of the disease. If your child starts to have periods of respiratory discomfort, and if these attacks are accompanied by audible wheezing sounds, place asthma high on the list of possible disorders.

During an asthma attack, a patient's respiratory rate—the number of respirations she takes per minute—will increase as the hours pass. At the same time, the depth of breathing—that is, the ability to take a full breath—will *decrease.* This is another indication that an attack is worsening.

During an asthma attack, bronchospasm and narrowing of the airways make it progressively more difficult for the child to exhale (usually inhaling is not a problem). Because of progressively worsening bronchial obstruction air becomes "trapped" in the balloon-like air sacs, which eventually causes the lungs to swell and the chest to expand. Children who suffer from severe and continual asthmatic episodes sometimes develop a chest abnormality known as "pigeon breast deformity." (If you can picture a pigeon with his chest puffed out, you can visualize how the chest of a severely asthmatic child may sometimes appear.)

Parents will find that children commonly suffer from asthma attacks at night. This may result from the fact that lying in a horizontal sleeping position causes mucus secretions to accumulate in the lungs. Or it may be due to the decreased production of cortisone in the child's system while he is asleep. Whatever the case, if your child is having problems with nocturnal attacks, it is a good idea to always have the proper medications on hand *before* local pharmacies close down for the evening.

Recognizing and Assessing an Asthma Emergency

At the beginning of any attack, notice that your child is breathing mainly by means of the chest muscles. As the attack progresses and as breathing becomes more labored, both the abdominal and the upper chest and neck muscles may join in the process, and eventually the spaces between the ribs, the bottom of the rib cage, and the area above the collarbones will all appear to be sucked in with every breath. These movements of the thorax are called "retractions" and are an indication that the patient's respiratory distress is increasing. When retractions are noted, which means the child is working harder to breathe, it is time to be in contact with your doctor.

Many children, especially younger ones, also complain of abdominal distress during asthma attacks. This problem develops for several reasons. First, due to downward pressure of the diaphragm caused by air trapped in the lungs, the stomach is squeezed in an unaccustomed manner, in some cases causing a whopping stomach ache. Second, many young children swallow excessive amounts of air during an attack; the stomach becomes accordingly distended and exerts pressure on the nerves, which in turn produce sharp abdominal pains. Though the child may be in acute misery from these cramps, they are rarely dangerous. However, do not ignore these symptoms. Third, many children swallow large amounts of mucus during an attack, which in turn produce significant abdominal irritation. As the asthma symptoms are brought under control, all these abdominal complaints will slowly subside.

During an attack, a child's heart and lungs work extraordinarily hard. As a result, heart rate is greatly accelerated. A rapid pulse does not usually mean trouble and is in fact to be expected whenever increased demands are made on the cardiac and respiratory systems. Consider what takes place after a session of intense physical activity—our hearts pound, breathing is rapid, the body sweats—and all these reactions are, of course, perfectly normal. You should realize that your child is experiencing the same physical sensations during an attack. Rarely if ever are cardiac problems or heart damage associated with such activity. Your child's pulse and respiratory rate will return to normal once the acute attack is brought under control.

If an attack is prolonged and no treatment is forthcoming, the child may begin to wheeze *less* than at the start of the episode. This situation generally takes many hours or even several days to develop. When it does occur—and if there is no corresponding ease of breathing to signify that the attack itself is subsiding—it is a serious warning sign. Repeat: *it is not a good sign.* If the chest becomes "silent," it develops because the bronchial air passageways are now so clogged with thickened, gluelike mucus that little or no air is moving through the lungs. The child's lungs are receiving inadequate amounts of air, and hence not enough oxygen is reaching the bloodstream. The process, in short, is a prelude to suffocation.

If the "silent" chest syndrome continues without treatment, or if the air passageways remain blocked for extensive periods of time, the child may also show signs of cyanosis, or lack of oxygen. Clinically, this condition can be recognized when the lips and fingernail beds turn a bluish color. The nail beds at the base of your child's fingernails are normally a lively pinkish-white color. During a severe asthmatic attack, lack of oxygen to the lungs turns them a morbid shade of blue, an indication that the attack is reaching the critical point.

Cyanosis requires *immediate* attention from a physician. REPEAT: IMMEDIATE! If your doctor is not available, get to the closest hospital emergency room without delay. The situation has reached the emergency stage. Suffocation is beginning!

Six Signs That Suggest a Trip to the Doctor*

- wheezing gets worse 1 to 3 hours after taking medicine
- child stops playing and cannot start again
- child has hard time breathing
- breathing gets faster 1 to 3 hours after taking medicine
- child has trouble walking or talking
- blue lips or fingernails—go immediately!

*SOURCE: C. H. Feldman and N. M. Clark, *Open Airways/Respiro Abierto: Asthma Self-Management Program,* National Heart, Lung, and Blood Institute, NIH Publication No. 84-2365.

During an asthma attack a child's rate of breathing will inevitably increase, and with each breath a measurable loss of water vapor follows. Children, especially very young ones, usually cannot tolerate eating or drinking during an attack, and these two factors, the loss of water vapor and the refusal or inability to take solids and liquids, frequently result in dehydration.

Loss of water from the lungs then causes mucus in the bronchi to become thick and gluelike, producing added blockage of the airways and hence increased respiratory discomfort. It is therefore vitally important that children be made to take some liquids during an asthmatic attack, even though eating and drinking are the farthest things from their minds, and that this be done by whatever methods are at hand. Don't be reluctant to offer soda, lemonade, water, anything that's wet. Some children like to suck on cracked ice. Others prefer warm liquids through a straw. Whatever you do, make sure that moderate amounts of fluids get *in*. If signs of dehydration are already present (symptoms include dry tongue, decrease in urination and a loss of the elastic quality of the skin), the child should receive immediate medical care.

There are a series of relatively simple medical observations that you as a parent can make to assess the seriousness of your child's condition.

Check respiration rates. How many breaths per minute are being taken? Using a watch, count the number of inhalations registered in thirty seconds. Double this number and you have the breaths-per-minute count. A normal rate, generally speaking, should be under 24 inhalations per minute (infants, as a rule, breathe somewhat faster—up to 30 breaths a minute). Each child's respiratory rate differs a bit, of course, so I suggest you determine this figure during an asthma-free period. Approach children while they are reading or watching TV, and record the number of breaths taken in a 30-second stretch (count the inhalation and exhalation as one complete breath). Then file this figure away for future reference. Measure it against your child's normal respiratory rate during the next asthmatic episode.

When does an increased breath count become cause for alarm? It is safe to say that more than 30 to 35 breaths per minute is increased. If this number climbs above 40 per minute, the danger zone has been entered: the child is obviously having respiratory distress and is working very hard to breathe. Seek medical help at once.

Check the pulse rate. How fast is the heart beating? The easiest pulses to count are located on the thumb side of the wrist (radial pulse), and along either side of the neck (carotid pulse). During an attack the neck vessels become especially prominent—you can sometimes see them throbbing during an attack —and are easy to locate. Count the number of beats at either of these pulse points for 15 seconds, multiply this number by four, and you have the pulse-per-minute rate.

A healthy and/or dangerous pulse rate differs for children according to their age, and again, infants have higher counts than older children. Pulse rates, in general, approach the danger zone when they climb above 120. If the count exceeds 125, talk to your doctor. It is also a good idea to keep a record of your child's resting pulse and respiration rate handy, even during asthma-free times. These statistics will help your physician gain a clear picture of the child's condition at your next visit. They can also be used as a baseline against which to gauge the seriousness of an attack when it occurs at home.

Each time your child has a substantial bout of asthma, check carefully for retractions. Retractions are sucking-in motions of the soft tissues located between, over and under the rib cage. Look carefully in the area above the collarbone for the presence of retractions. Are the movements confined to the abdominal and chest area? Your physician will want to know precisely where the retractions are located and how long they have been present.

Observe the nature of your child's cough. Though the noise of a loose rattle and associated mucus buildup may sound unpleasant, this very loose, loud quality is probably a positive sign. It is the body's method of clearing foreign matter out of the bronchial tree and moving mucus secretions from one area of the lung to another until they can be coughed out or swallowed. When mucus is expectorated, moreover, its color and texture offer critical clues to what is taking place in the lungs. Thin, clear and whitish mucus is, generally speaking, a good sign. Mucus that is discolored or coughed up in firm plugs indicates that an infection may be present or an attack has been going on for a fairly long time.

If the nature of the child's cough changes from loose and wet to persistent, dry and hacking, this means the attack is worsening. Speak with the doctor right away.

Is your child able to retain food, fluids and medication? If not, be aware that nausea and vomiting may occur. For a number of reasons, it is always important to determine the cause and be able to control these symptoms.

Young children frequently will vomit as a result of having swallowed large amounts of mucus, a substance highly irritating to the lining of the stomach. They may also develop this symptom when the stomach becomes distended and swollen due to large amounts of swallowed air. Downward pressure of the diaphragm on the stomach is another possible explanation for vomiting.

The bronchodilator medications used to control the asthma attack can sometimes trigger vomiting, either because of gastric irritation or as a toxic symptom of theophylline overdosage.

As a rule, during an attack children feel better after they have vomited the large amounts of irritating mucus which accumulate in the stomach. However, if the vomiting continues, call the doctor. Be prepared to tell the physician how frequently the child has vomited and to describe the regurgitated material.

Never allow an attack of asthma to go on too long before consulting a physician. And don't suppose that this particular episode will be shorter than the last: there is no reason to make such an assumption; the opposite case can just as easily be true. Remember, *the longer an asthmatic attack is allowed to continue without treatment, the more difficult it will be to control once medical advice is sought.* Get help early, before things get worse.

Some Significant Facts about Asthma You Should Know

Asthma and the emotions Despite a lingering popular notion that asthma is an "emotional disease," instances of asthma originating exclusively or even primarily because of psychological causes are, in my experience, unusual. This is not to suggest that a child who experiences recurrent asthmatic episodes may not develop an emotional response to the condition, or that stressful psychological situations do not occasionally worsen the disease. Such emotional or psychological reactions are, however, *secondary* to the underlying condition itself. They are, so to speak, side effects and are rarely the actual cause of the attack. According to what is known today, asthma is first and foremost a physiologic disorder. It is *not* the result of an emotional disorder.

All the more reason for parents to be aware of the child who recognizes that his asthma can be fashioned into an emotional weapon that can be used to manipulate Mom and Dad.

It is risky business to let asthmatic children get away with behavior for which their nonasthmatic siblings would be immediately punished. While it is obviously important to appreciate the psychological trauma severe asthma can cause, in most cases it is inadvisable to hold on to the old-fashioned notions that it is the child's "unhappiness" or "maladjustment" that is at the root of the ailment. For parents who persist in perpetuating this no-win scenario, and for children who encourage it, a physician's referral to a psychiatrist or psychologist may be in the best interests of everyone concerned.

Can a child outgrow asthma? There is simply no solid evidence to support the notion that the hormonal changes occurring during puberty will have any effect on your child's asthma condition. To the inevitable question all parents ask, "Will my child outgrow asthma?" the most honest answer I or any other allergist can give is "No one knows." Certainly some children appear to get better as they grow older. But whether *your* child will lose *his* particular symptoms, no one can tell.

One generalization can be made: Approximately one-third of all asthmatic children will improve as they grow older; one-third will get worse; one-third will stay the same. Those who improve generally do so by adolescence. Statistics are well and good when talking to a large audience, of course, but I realize it is a relatively unsatisfactory response in a one-on-one discussion. With all due apologies, it is simply the best that can be done given the present state of our knowledge.

Asthma and your child's heart Though children with severe asthma will often puff and pant, turn red and white in the face and go through such contortions during an attack that parents fear for their very lives, it should be stressed that asthma rarely causes damage to the heart. Only under the most unusual circumstances can it cause permanent changes in any organ, including the lungs.

Exercise-induced asthma Physical exertion is often the stimulus that triggers wheezing in asthmatic children. In fact, there are some youngsters who *only* wheeze after periods of strenuous physical exertion, and whose lungs are otherwise normal. This particular type of asthma is called *exercise-induced asthma,* abbreviated as EIA.

Running, football, soccer and basketball are well-known EIA triggers, while cycling, tennis and especially swimming are less likely to bring on attacks. We do know that if exertion takes place in a cool, dry atmosphere, wheezing is more likely to occur than when the weather is warm and humid. In other words, your child may have no problems playing actively during the summer months, but the same activity performed on a windy, wintery day will rapidly produce EIA.

Typically, the child with EIA develops wheezing at the *end* of an exercise period, and the symptoms disappear within 30 to 90 minutes. A small number of children with EIA will also experience a delayed onset of symptoms, beginning four to eight hours after the exercise has ended. This delayed-response pattern tends to produce more severe wheezing than the immediate response and should therefore be carefully monitored. Fortunately, the use of specific asthma medications, aerosol beta-adrenergic agents and cromolyn sodium in particular, given a few minutes before exertion will usually keep even severe cases of EIA under control. We will discuss these medications shortly.

Diagnosing Your Child's Asthma: How It's Done

Wheezing is probably an indication of asthma, but not invariably. In attempting to diagnose the cause of a wheeze, the first thing you must do is become familiar with asthma's wheeze-causing "look-alikes," which at first glance sound and look like asthma, but stem from entirely different causes. Before taking your wheezing child to a specialist, review the following conditions. They will help you and your doctor zero in on the cause of your child's wheezing.

In early infancy, nasal obstruction or congestion can cause a child to produce wheeze-like sounds. These sounds actually originate in the nasal passageways, not in the lungs, and have nothing to do with asthma. In most cases, careful observation by the parents will help differentiate between the two conditions. At times it is difficult without a stethoscope to decide where the wheezing sound originates. A visit to the doctor is recommended if symptoms persist.

In certain very young children there may be an abnormality of the trachea called tracheomalacia. Here the trachea's cartilage rings partially collapse each time a child inhales, creating a wheezing-type sound in the process. Ordinarily, as the child grows older the cartilage rings become stiffer, and the condition corrects itself.

Less common are the so-called webs, rings or slings which exert pressure on the trachea and major bronchi, and which are formed from anatomical abnormalities of the major blood vessels near the heart. These rings occasionally become so prominent that they partially block the trachea or the esophagus, producing asthma-like symptoms. This condition requires surgical correction.

Between the ages of one and three, random objects inadvertently swallowed by a child often prove to be the true cause behind respiratory symptoms, especially if wheezing sounds are localized to only one side of the chest. Small, easily swallowable items such as rings, coins, blades of grass, small toys and pebbles are fished out of children every day of the year, and all can produce bronchospasm. The sudden onset of respiratory distress with wheezing should be a signal to get your child to a doctor or an emergency room.

Childhood infections such as croup, bronchitis and pneumonia may induce wheezing symptoms parents mistakenly identify as asthma. The same is true with bronchiolitis, a viral respiratory disorder that involves the smaller parts of the breathing tubes and which generally strikes infants. Some children who have recurring attacks of bronchiolitis are actually demonstrating the first stage of a true asthmatic condition. This pattern tends to be especially true if there is a positive history of asthma or allergy in the family. Your doctor will fill you in on the details. If your child has any respiratory symptoms such as persistent cough, wheeze or shortness of breath, discuss the situation with your doctor.

In addition to the preceding conditions there are a number of other situations in which asthma-like symptoms may be present. These include: anatomic abnormalities of the trachea and bronchial tubes, the rare presence of a cyst or tumor within the respiratory tract and such medical conditions as cystic fibrosis or tuberculosis. Exposure to toxic chemicals and air pollutants can certainly cause respiratory distress with shortness of breath and wheezing. In order to diagnose most of these conditions a doctor will have to examine your child.

Once you have reason to believe that your child suffers from asthma, the single most important service you can render an allergist is to prepare a thoughtful, complete medical history and to present it to the doctor at the first visit. Briefly speaking, the most important points to cover include:

- when your child's symptoms began
- frequency of the child's attacks
- particular situations that trigger episodes
- medical measures that have been taken in the past
- types of medication used
- the child's typical level of activities

The more information you supply the specialist at the time of the initial visit, the more specific will be his diagnosis and his recommendations. For more details on preparing a child's personal medical history, see the checklist on page 16.

Specific Diagnostic Tests for Asthma

After examining your child and checking her medical history, the doctor may wish to run several diagnostic tests to determine if asthma is the correct diagnosis. Though the majority of tests used for this purpose have been described on pages 22–30, let's review the common ones and add a few that have not yet been mentioned:

X-ray   If there has been a significant increase in a child's respiratory symptoms, if there has been an obvious change in their pattern and frequency, if the child has suffered from breathing problems for a prolonged period of time, and if no chest X-rays have been taken to date, X-ray studies will probably be ordered. They are not a standard procedure, however, and will only be called for when the above conditions prevail.

EKG (Electrocardiogram)   Usually an EKG is requested only when there is a history of heart problems or when the physical exam turns up evidence of possible cardiac trouble, such as a heart murmur. If neither of these conditions is present, I would advise that you inquire directly as to why the EKG has been ordered. Presumably your physician has specific reasons, but you as a parent are entitled to know about them. The test itself is neither painful nor harmful and may provide the doctor with important data. If a child has suffered from extremely severe asthma and has been repeatedly hospitalized for this condition, the doctor will attempt to get as much information as possible concerning the child's cardiovascular and respiratory systems; then an EKG will probably be ordered.

Allergy tests   These include the direct and indirect skin tests discussed at length on pages 25–28. If any of these tests are positive, it does not necessarily mean that the allergen responsible for the response is causing asthma, only that it is now a strong possible suspect. After the test results are obtained, the doctor must by means of observation, analysis of the personal medical history, and a synthesis of all that is known concerning the child's condition, decide whether a clinical relationship really does exist between asthma and the positive test results.

Blood tests   Several may be ordered. These include the CBC or complete blood count (see page 22) and the IgE level determination test (see page 23). Another, the quantitative immunoglobulins test (see page 22), is requested mainly for patients demonstrating a pattern of frequent severe bacterial infections. If, in fact, abnormally low levels of certain protective antibodies are found in the bloodstream, patients may require special treatment against such infections.

Sputum test   Microscopic studies of sputum or mucus secretions coughed up from the lungs during an attack are rarely done on a routine basis in the case of asthma. It is often difficult to get an adequate specimen from younger children (just ask a two-year-old to cough and spit up on demand), and the laboratory facilities needed to carry out the test may not be readily available.

Bronchial inhalation challenge tests An allergen believed to be the cause of a child's asthma is inhaled directly in aerosol form, and the patient is observed to see if any signs of an allergic response develop. (Sometimes methacoline or histamine are used in place of specific allergens, both of which trigger wheezing attacks in susceptible subjects but leave nonasthmatics unaffected.) The metacholine and histamine challenge can be used as a differential test to decide if a patient really is asthmatic. Inhalation challenge tests are done in a hospital or office with a physician in constant attendance so that when and if severe wheezing develops, the appropriate medicine can then be quickly administered. If a child reacts to a specific allergen during the test with changes in pulmonary function or with obvious clinical asthma symptoms, then the diagnosis of allergic asthma is confirmed.

Challenge tests are done infrequently and only when the diagnosis is a difficult one. The test has hazards built into it: provoking an asthmatic attack always creates the possibility of severe symptoms developing, though with proper precautions this procedure can be of great help and provide information essential for the management of the child's condition. If your child is scheduled to take such a test, it is in her best interest to describe beforehand how and where the procedure will be done and that she will not have to remain in the hospital after the test is completed.

Pulmonary function study As soon as a child is old enough to cooperate fully with a physician—usually around the age of five or six—pulmonary function studies will be ordered (see page 29). Younger children sometimes can be tested with a simple device called a peak flow meter. There is good evidence to suggest that any child with chronic asthma symptoms should be monitored at home with daily peak flow meter determinations. These tests are done with a variety of mechanical devices, both large and small. They are designed to measure the abnormalities typically found in the lungs of a child with chronic asthma and to determine how well the child's lungs are actually working. By and large, this test is quick and painless. The child breathes into a mechanical device and the strength and quality of each breath is recorded, measured and then evaluated by the allergist. Most children with asthma will demonstrate some degree of functional abnormality during these studies, even when no signs of breathing difficulty are evident.

Arterial blood gas determination In severely asthmatic patients, especially those who have experienced long-term, persistent wheezing, the oxygen level in the bloodstream becomes significant: a sizable decrease in this level, or an increase in the CO_2 (carbon dioxide) level of the blood may warn of impending respiratory failure. When either of these dangerous conditions is noted, very aggressive treatment will be called for, including the administration of oxygen and intravenous fluids and the use of bronchodilators and cortisone. Arterial blood gas studies are almost always performed in an emergency room or in another hospital setting.

Treating Your Child's Asthma

Environmental Control

The first and perhaps easiest way to treat an asthmatic child is simply to remove the child from the source of the symptoms. If this maneuver is impossible, then the child's environment can be manipulated in such a way that exposure to particular allergens will be minimized. If you avoid exposure, you can avoid symptoms.

If, for example, it is known that contact with an animal or a certain food triggers symptoms, everyone involved should realize that the child must be kept away from these allergens.

Simple. But this fact is not as obvious to some as logic might dictate. In my medical practice I am constantly asked by the parents of animal-sensitive children for permission to bring a pet into the home. Despite the child's known susceptibilities to animal dander and despite an observable one-on-one relationship between contact with the allergen and an allergic response, some parents continue to believe that the child will somehow muddle through it all or that the allergy will magically disappear on its own.

But it usually doesn't. In fact, it should be obvious to parents that if a specific substance or circumstance triggered an allergic problem yesterday, then this agent will most likely do the same thing today, perhaps with even greater severity. Until you know for sure that a child has gotten over his sensitivity to a particular allergen, keep that particular allergen and that particular child very far apart.

CHECKLIST OF POTENTIAL ALLERGENS FOR ASTHMATIC CHILDREN TO AVOID
What allergenic agents trigger asthma in children? What can be done to minimize or neutralize their effects? Here is a representative checklist:

Certain animals. Dogs, cats, birds and rabbits in particular are primary causes of allergic asthma. Better tolerated are guinea pigs, hamsters, reptiles and all varieties of fish. If hairy, furry or feathered pets must for whatever reason be kept in the home, they should be banished from the child's bedroom, and preferably from his general area of the house. If possible, keep these animals restricted to one section of the home, ideally in those areas most easily cleaned—i.e., rooms free of dander-gathering fabrics, rugs, upholstered furniture and heavy drapes. An even better solution is to keep the pet permanently out-of-doors.

Feathers. These are found primarily in bedding, sleeping bags and stuffed furniture. It is a good policy to keep all allergic asthmatic children away from down and from all types of birds. Feather-sensitive children can usually wear down vests or outerwear, but they will find it difficult to sleep under a down comforter *all night* without experiencing symptoms. In other words, the intensity of the exposure determines if symptoms will or will not develop.

Wool. Found in carpets, blankets and in woolen clothing such as shirts, dresses, socks, scarfs, etc. I am often asked whether or not an allergic asthmatic child can wear a woolen coat. The answer is usually yes, except children who develop skin rashes from wool.

Dusty environments. Shun them. Dust is both an allergen and a just-plain-irritating substance. Exposure to a room full of dust can cause nasal congestion, sneezing and for many children an asthma attack. To help combat irritating inhalants, filtering devices can be used to clean the air of dust, cigarette smoke, pollens and a variety of other allergens. See pages 130–132 for detailed information.

Molds. Household areas such as attics, crawl spaces and cellars are predisposed to mold growth and should be avoided. In many cases dampness will cause asthma and so will molds. The combination of the two can be a disaster.

Controlled humidity. During the winter, when heating units make homes arid and hot, it is best to keep the indoor relative humidity between 35 and 45 percent, even if an electronic humidifier must be installed to do the trick (see page 130).

Heating systems. Be aware of the effects of household heating systems. The worst from the point of view of an asthmatic child is the forced-air type. The hot billows of bone-dry air that pour out of these units stir up room dust like small cyclones and tend to dry out the mucous membranes of the throat. Steam radiators are something of an improvement, and baseboard heating is better still. Excellent, though most expensive, is radiant electric heat. Now that I have condemned forced-air heating, however, it should be noted that a forced-air system supplied with a built-in humidifier and an electronic filter is a wonderful setup for environmentally controlled living. In fact, a system of this kind is probably the very best of all possible heating arrangements in a household with an allergic or asthmatic family member.

Air conditioning. In most instances, air conditioning is an aid for allergy and asthma sufferers. The one exception is the case of the child who is especially sensitive to abrupt changes of air temperature and whose breathing becomes suddenly labored whenever she enters an air-conditioned house on a hot summer day. In such instances air conditioning is obviously more of a liability than an asset and should not be used. Do not make the mistake of thinking that an air conditioner filters the air of all undesirable particles. It doesn't, at least not to any dependable degree. To remove ultrafine particles typical of smoke, pollen, molds and other minute allergens, special air filtration systems will almost always be necessary (see page 132).

Asthma Medications for Your Child: As Complete a Survey as You'll Ever Need

First, a word of warning: If your child suffers from bronchial asthma, do not self-medicate him; use only drugs prescribed by a trained physician.

This said, we can get to the business of describing the most commonly prescribed asthma medicines. While it may seem to the bewildered parent that there are an endless number of these medications, they are, in fact, rather limited. All the asthma drugs you may have run across through the years are simply varieties and brand names of the same small number of drug families.

BRONCHODILATORS   *Theophylline*   Sold under a number of brand names, the bronchodilator theophylline has been in use for the treatment of bronchial asthma since 1937. In 1983, its national sales approached $120 million (which gives you some idea of asthma's prevalence in this country), and in the United States it is now the single most commonly prescribed antiasthma medication. Chances are that if your child has asthma some form of theophylline will at some point be included in his asthma-management program. Some of the more popular commercial forms include Slo-Phyllin, Theo-Dur, Theophyl, Slo-bid, Bronkodyl, Theolair and Aminophylline. A more definitive list can be found in Table 3.

How does it work? In many ways. Most importantly, it relaxes the smooth muscle surrounding the bronchi or breathing tubes, thereby reducing obstruction of the lungs. It also stimulates the cilia, those millions of tiny hairlike follicles lining the airways which serve to propel mucus up and out of the lungs, keeping the respiratory system clean of excess secretions and cellular debris. Theophylline also stimulates the central nervous system during asthmatic episodes, specifically the respiratory center. Lastly, there is some evidence that theophylline improves the muscle function of both the diaphragm and various other respiratory muscles, thus strengthening the lungs during an attack. In all, a highly useful and efficacious medication.

For many years theophylline was not prescribed for children, because of inadequate information regarding its appropriate dose and an increased number of asthma deaths that resulted from overdoses, mainly by the inappropriate use of aminophylline suppositories. Over the past decade or so our knowledge of theophylline's chemistry and our ability to monitor theophylline levels in the blood with precision have improved to such an extent that this drug is currently considered agent number one for the treatment of childhood asthma.

This increase in our knowledge does not mean, of course, that theophylline is without potential problems.

Limitations and side effects Theophylline is a highly effective bronchodilator for most children, but not for all. Some simply cannot tolerate it; others have such an erratic metabolism that it becomes almost impossible to regulate dosages. Certain children tolerate the drug quite nicely in such low doses as to perhaps not be clinically effective.

In general, it can be said that a majority of theophylline's side effects stem from too high a dose, not from the action of the drug itself. Parents are advised to become familiar with these side effects (as well as the side effects of any other medication your child is taking), and to carefully describe any questionable symptoms to your doctor. The signs and symptoms to watch for with theophylline overdose consist of the following:

Nausea, loss of appetite, vomiting and heartburn.

Rapid heartbeat, palpitations and in a few very rare cases irregular heart rhythms. This in no way means that theophylline causes cardiac problems or that it damages the heart. Symptoms vanish as soon as the medication is stopped.

Headaches, restlessness and insomnia. While it has not been proven, there is also a possibility that some children taking theophylline on a daily schedule may experience a decrease in their ability to concentrate. If it should occur, stopping the drug eliminates this problem.

Hyperactivity. Some children become hyperactive even though the amount of theophylline in their bloodstream is well within the normal treatment range. Such patients are simply unable to tolerate this medicine regardless of the amount administered.

Quite a list. But remember, these symptoms only develop in a small minority of children who are on theophylline. If you are aware of the potential problems, then the medicine can be discontinued or changed at the earliest signs of trouble.

Still, there are youngsters who suffer some side effects of theophylline even when the drug is administered in appropriate dosages. Headaches may occur, as well as heartburn, nausea, hyperactivity. If these reactions continue, it means that your child's body chemistry is simply not compatible with the drug. If the dose is readjusted several times and there is still no improvement, a new medication must be tried. It must, however, be stressed once again that most children when given a carefully regulated dose of theophylline can take it for long periods of time without developing adverse reactions of any kind.

Clearance rate Many conditions such as age, weight and diet affect the way a child metabolizes any medication. These conditions will cause the body either to increase the speed at which the medicine is used up or to slow it down. The measurement of how rapidly the body consumes a specific drug is known as the *clearance rate,* and this rate will vary from child to child. As a rule, children metabolize theophylline more quickly than adults and require more of the substance per pound of body weight. Table 1 illustrates how clearance rates work with regard to several critical variables.

What exactly does the clearance rate tell us about the way a child reacts to theophylline and to medications in general? A *decreased* clearance rate means that the drug is remaining in the child's system longer than was expected and that it may be reaching a toxic level in the blood with resultant side

Table 1.   Theophylline Blood Levels

**Factors That Can Increase
Circulating Levels of Theophylline**

High carbohydrate diet

Drugs: Cimetidine (Tagamet)

   Clindamycin

   Erythromycin estolate

   Troleandomycin (TAD)

Heart failure

Kidney failure

Liver failure

Viral infections

Pulmonary edema

**Factors That Can Decrease
Circulating Levels of Theophylline**

High protein diet

Charcoal-broiled foods

Smoking tobacco or marijuana

Young children (under age five) rapidly metabolize theophylline. Therefore they require higher doses based on their weight than older children or adolescents.

effects. An *increased* rate causes the drug to be used up faster than was expected, lowering the amount of drug in the bloodstream so that it fails to produce the anticipated therapeutic effects.

There are, in addition to the conditions listed above, children who by nature are either rapid or slow metabolizers of theophylline. This means that for these children it will be necessary to closely monitor the amount of theophylline in the blood. Actually, any child who will be taking a theophylline preparation on a long-term daily basis will require periodic theophylline blood level determinations.

Dosage Naturally, it is the doctor's responsibility to prescribe the appropriate dose of theophylline, but as a parent you must have a general understanding of how the doctor arrives at the theophylline dose for your child.

In the case of theophylline, the dose is decided by two factors, both of which have a strong bearing on the way the child utilizes the drug: age and weight. Table 2 provides a guide to dosage strengths. Use it to determine whether or not your child is receiving medication within the range appropriate for age and weight. If something seems out of the ordinary, do not come to hasty conclusions until you speak with your physician—it must be stressed that the figures in Table 2 are based on averages and are not chiseled in stone. Most likely it will turn out that there is sound method to the doctor's decisions.

Blood tests Ideally, all children who are taking theophylline regularly should have a periodic (every six months) blood test done in order to determine if they are receiving the correct dose of medicine. If a youngster will be on theophylline for only a relatively short time (less than two weeks) and he is doing well on the medication, there is no need for a theophylline level determination.

The main reason for doing this test is to let everyone know if the prescribed dose of theophylline is providing the patient with a therapeutic blood level. The optimal effective level of theophylline in the circulation is between 10 and 20 micrograms per milliliter of blood. Levels above this range are frequently associated with signs and symptoms of theophylline toxicity. When the circulating level is under 10 micrograms per milliliter, the bronchodilating effect of theophylline is definitely decreased, though I have had patients who are clinically well with theophylline levels of less than 10 micrograms.

Table 2.   *Theophylline Dose Recommendations*

Age or Predisposing Condition	Milligrams of Theophylline per Kilogram of Body Weight* per Twenty-Four-Hour Period
Children	
12 months–9 years	18–20
9–16 years Young adult smokers	16
Adults	
Healthy, nonsmoking	10
Over 50 years with heart condition	6
Children or Adults	
Congestive heart failure Liver disease	2.4

NOTE: It is always safer to begin treatment with a dose approximately two-thirds of the recommended amount and gradually increase the dose to the recommended level. For any patient who will be maintained on a constant regimen of theophylline, it is important to periodically check the theophylline blood level.

*The proper dose of theophylline should be based on a person's *ideal* or *lean* body weight.

How do these tests work? Most likely your doctor will want to check the drug's peak level first. This test is performed when the maximum amount of theophylline is circulating in the system: one to two hours after a short-acting form of the drug has been administered; four to five hours after a long-acting or sustained-release form is used. A small amount of blood is taken from a vein or a finger stick to be analyzed.

If major problems exist with regulating the theophylline dose, it may also be necessary to check the trough, or lowest blood level. This level is reached just before the effects of the drug are wearing off when the patient is ready for a new dose (this can be anywhere from six to eight or even twelve hours after the medicine has been administered). It is unusual to get a trough level determination, and in practice it is usually only necessary to check the peak level.

The concept of therapeutic drug monitoring—checking the amount of medicine circulating in the bloodstream—is an accepted practice in all fields of medicine, but as with any new medical procedure, costs are high and widespread availability of the tests is still limited. Both these problems, happily, are currently being solved. Specifically for theophylline there are now at least two reasonably priced systems available which allow physicians to check a patient's blood levels in the office. I believe that within the next five years there will be test kits available for checking theophylline levels in the home.

Threading your way through the theophylline maze In 1985 there were over sixty-four different entries under *theophylline* in *A Physician's Desk Reference.* This number is growing every year, and it becomes increasingly confusing for both physician and patient to decide which brand, which type, which form is the best for a particular case. The problem can be somewhat simplified by adding a few facts to what you already know about theophylline.

Until ten years ago, theophylline was prepared commercially in combination with a variety of other drugs. For many asthmatic patients these combination preparations were quite effective, but for others, especially children, they were poorly tolerated and side effects abounded. What's more, if patients needed an increased dose of theophylline, it was necessary to take elevated amounts of all the other drugs as well, as they came together in fixed drug combinations. Today we know that fixed drug combinations are certainly not appropriate preparations for treating childhood asthma symptoms. In those situations when a patient on theophylline requires additional medication to control her asthma, a second bronchodilator preparation can be added as a supplement. This is a benefit, of course, for when drugs are prescribed individually rather than in fixed combinations the doctor maintains control over the appropriate doses of each, gaining the best results while minimizing side effects.

Theophylline comes in two basic forms: short acting and long acting or sustained release. The short-acting forms are available in liquid, tablets, chewable tablets or capsules. They are usually taken once every six hours and reach a peak level in the bloodstream within one to two hours.

The long-acting or sustained-release preparations are available as tablets, capsules, and the so-called sprinkle forms. Sprinkles are capsules filled with hundreds of tiny beads that are shaken directly onto foods such as applesauce or whipped topping and are then swallowed along with the food. Do not let the child chew these granules. They taste terrible and chewing will destroy their long-acting properties.

For an acute wheezing attack, the short-acting forms of theophylline provide the quickest relief. After 48 hours on a short-acting preparation a child can be switched to a sustained-release theophylline preparation that has to be taken only every 12 hours. The advantage of sustained-release theophylline is that the intervals between doses are longer than with the short-acting forms (the short-acting form is administered every 6 hours). With sustained-release theophylline it thus becomes unnecessary to wake children at night or to interrupt their studies at school to give the medication.

Stick as close as possible to a regular schedule for the administration of theophylline. Dosage times should become as familiar and habitual to your child's daily living rhythms as lunchtime or bedtime. If for whatever reason a child does miss her dose, do *not* make it up by giving a double dose next time. The treatment range and the toxic range of theophylline are rather close, and too much given at one time can easily cause side effects.

Theophylline is such a bitter-tasting chemical that drug manufacturers have found it impossible to produce a truly palatable liquid form. Children usually down the pills and the capsules and especially the sprinkles without a major struggle, but even adults cannot tolerate the liquid. This is especially problematic in the case of very young children who have difficulty swallowing pills and who must take the liquid form or none at all. In such cases, remember that the more concentrated the liquid, the less medicine your child must swallow (strengths are listed on the bottle). You might also try making the potion more acceptable by mixing it with a strong sweetener. Parents have reported some measure of success with standard seductions such as maple syrup.

Table 3 is by no means all inclusive, and there are certainly other satisfactory forms of theophylline on the market. I've listed these particular brands simply because they have proven themselves effective in my own practice.

Other potential dangers Though theophylline is ordinarily a safe drug, as with all medications, misuse can cause trouble and even danger. The most important thing for parents to realize in this regard is that *under no circumstances should they attempt to medicate a child with theophylline* without medical guidance. Occasionally parents with more than one asthmatic child will have a surplus of the drug on hand and they will randomly give Johnny's medication to Suzie during an attack. THIS IS A SERIOUS MISTAKE. The precise theophylline dose, as we have seen, is a critical factor in treatment, not only to insure the best clinical response but to avoid potentially dangerous side effects.

Beta-adrenergic agents (or drugs) Beta-adrenergic agents are a group of drugs chemically related to epinephrine (Adrenalin) which, like theophylline, belong to the bronchodilator drug family. During the past two decades, chem-

Table 3.   Commonly Prescribed Theophylline Preparations

Brand Name	Strength (in milligrams)	Color	Usual Dosage Interval (in hours)	Amount of Theophylline (in milligrams)	Scored Tablet Available
Short-Acting Capsules					
Bronkodyl	100	Brown/white	6–8	100	No
	200	Green/white		200	No
Elixophyllin	100	White	6–8	100	No
	200	Red		200	No
Quibron -300*	300	Yellow/white	6–8	300	No
Short-Acting Tablets					
Slo-Phyllin	100	White	6	100	Yes
	200	White		200	Yes
Theolair	125	White	6	125	No
	250	White		250	No
Theophyl chewable	100	White	6	100	Yes (in quarters)
Long-Acting Capsules					
Aerolate	65	Red/white	12	65	No
	130	Red/white		130	No
	260	Red/white		260	No
Slo-Phyllin gyrocaps	60	White	8–12	60	No
	125	Brown		125	No
	250	Purple		250	No
Theophyl-SR	125	Yellow	8–12	125	No
	250	Green		250	No
Long-Acting "Sprinkle" Capsules					
Slo-bid gyrocaps	50	Clear/white	8–12	50	No
	100	Clear/white		100	No
	200	White/clear		200	No
	300	White/clear		300	No
Theo-Dur	50	White/black	8–12	50	No

Table 3. (Continued)

Brand Name	Strength (in milli-grams)	Color	Usual Dosage Interval (in hours)	Amount of Theophyl-line (in milli-grams)	Scored Tablet Available
Theo-Dur	50	White/black	8–12	50	No
	75	White/green		75	No
	125	White/red		125	No
	200	White/blue		200	No
Long-Acting Tablets					
Labid	250	White	12	250	Yes
Theo-Dur	100	White	12	100	Yes
	200	White		200	Yes
	300	White		300	Yes
Theolair-SR	200	White	12	200	Yes
	250	White		250	Yes
	300	White		300	Yes
	500	White		500	Yes
Liquid					
Bronkodyl elixir†	80/15 ml.	Red	6	26/5 ml.	—
Quibron	150/15 ml.	Pale yellow	6	50/5 ml.	—
Slo-Phyllin -80	80/15 ml.	Orange	6	26/5 ml.	—
Theolair	80/15 ml.	Clear	6	26/5 ml.	—
Somophyllin	90/5 ml.	Clear	6	90/5 ml.	—

NOTE: All medications are 100 percent theophylline unless otherwise indicated.

*Quibron-300 is compounded with guaifenesin.

†Bronkodyl elixir contains 20 percent alcohol.

ists and clinical pharmacologists have produced a constant stream of these preparations, so that today the beta-adrenergic class of bronchodilators represent the fastest-growing area of asthma pharmacotherapy.

Side effects Skeletal-muscle tremor is perhaps the most frequent side effect of these drugs. In a child a common indication of this side effect is an obvious worsening of penmanship, sometimes clearly visible trembling of the hands. Teachers will complain that a child who has been an attentive pupil now can't seem to sit still. Fortunately, most children will tolerate this symptom, and within five to seven days the shakiness will disappear. This problem appears in only 10 to 25 percent of children who are started on this class of bronchodilators.

Other less frequent complaints include rapid heartbeat (tachycardia) and bouts of insomnia. Parents occasionally report that their child has become extremely hyper while being treated, and occasionally I hear of a usually well-behaved child suddenly acting off the wall when using these medicines. In such cases the medication must of course be adjusted or discontinued.

What follows is a discussion of the most commonly used preparations.

Epinephrine (Adrenalin) This drug is probably the single most effective medication doctors have for the treatment of acute bronchial asthma. Its main disadvantage is that it must be given by injection, a process which requires a visit to the doctor's office or to a hospital emergency room.

When administered early in the course of an asthmatic episode, epinephrine sometimes will completely stop an attack. More often it significantly improves symptoms, decreasing both wheezing and cough. This response usually lasts from one to four hours before the symptoms recur: remember, bronchodilators only control the symptoms; they cannot cure the disease.

For persistent wheezing, epinephrine shots can be repeated at fifteen- to thirty-minute intervals for a total of three doses. If the symptoms do not respond to this treatment, the patient's condition is termed *status asthmaticus,* a situation calling for immediate admission to the hospital. Status asthmaticus is a condition of persistent asthma unresponsive to the usual methods of treatment. We will discuss status asthmaticus in greater detail on page 101.

There are two forms of epinephrine in common use. The first is an aqueous (water) preparation that is short acting. Its dose is determined by the age and the weight of the child, but no more than 0.3 cc should be administered in a single dose.

The second form is a long-acting aqueous suspension called Sus-Phrine. As a rule it is prescribed only after the child has been given the short-acting form several times with positive results and with no serious side effects. Once Sus-Phrine is given, no additional epinephrine should be administered for at least four to six hours. The dose of Sus-Phrine, like the short-acting form, is based on child's age and weight. The maximum pediatric dose is 0.15 cc.

There are other adrenergic drugs listed here. Some of them are older and less commonly prescribed than epinephrine. Others are simply not as effective or are so new that the verdict on them is not yet in.

• *Ephedrine* The oldest of the oral adrenergic bronchodilators, today this drug is used infrequently. The new beta-adrenergic agents are more effective and cause fewer side effects.

• *Isoproterenol* Commonly known as Isuprel, this drug stimulates both the heart and lungs, sometimes to such a degree that the rapid heartbeat becomes a distressing side effect. It is most effective when used as an aerosol. Though a standby for years as a proven asthma medication, Isuprel has a comparatively short duration of action when measured against the newer, more effective drugs. There is a liquid oral preparation of Isuprel on the market that is metabolized and inactivated in the stomach so quickly that it is ineffective. Under no circumstances would I recommend it.

• *Isoetharine* This drug is marketed either as Bronkosol, to be used with an aerosol compressor pump, or as Bronkometer, which is a hand-held type of nebulizer called a metered dose inhaler (MDI). Isoetharine's duration of action, like that of Isuprel, is relatively short. On the positive side, it is somewhat less likely than Isuprel to cause heart palpitations.

• *Metaproterenol* This preparation, one of the newer beta-adrenergic bronchodilator medications, is sold under the brand names Alupent and Metaprel. It is available as a pill, liquid and in solution (Alupent) for use with an aerosol compressor pump or an MDI. Metaproterenol's period of symptom control generally lasts for three to six hours. While the oral forms are approved for use in children over the age of six and the aerosol forms are recommended for patients twelve and over, this drug has been used effectively for children much younger than the officially recommended age. Ultimately, the decision to use or not use metaproterenol for young children must rest with each individual physician.

• *Terbutaline* This drug, also known as Bricanyl and Brethine, is available as an MDI aerosol, as a solution for injection, and in 2.5- or 5-milligram tablets. Terbutaline is a very useful medication with a duration of action from four to eight hours; the FDA has recommended that in aerosol form it be used by children twelve years of age or older.

• *Albuterol* Marketed as Proventil or Ventolin, this drug is available in liquid, tablet and MDI form. It is probably the most effective beta-adrenergic aerosol medication available in the United States today; I have been extremely pleased with the good results patients have had when using it, especially the MDI form. The FDA has recommended that the MDI form be used in individuals twelve years of age or older.

While the usual recommended dose of albuterol is two puffs taken every six hours, there are certain situations in which the dosing interval can be reduced to once every four hours, or even less. Your doctor should review with you those special circumstances when it may be appropriate to use a MDI on a more frequent schedule.

A complete discussion with your doctor regarding the proper technique

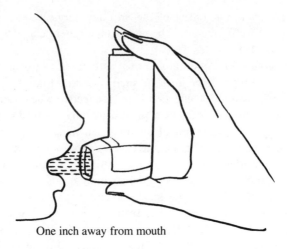

One inch away from mouth

Proper metered dose inhaler (MDI) position

for using the metered dose inhaler should take place at the time the medication is prescribed.

The spray released when you discharge a gas-propelled, hand-held metered dose inhaler leaves the mouthpiece at approximately sixty to seventy miles per hour. In other words, the medicine doesn't take very long to reach its destination, and if your child does not accurately synchronize her inhalation with the spray, very little of the medicine will ever reach her lungs. When you visit the doctor ask for specific directions on how to use this device. Go over these directions several times.

For handy reference, here are the fundamentals regarding MDI use.

1. Shake the inhaler for several seconds before using. The part that holds the medicine, the canister, must be held upright and positioned *above* the mouthpiece during use.
2. It is best to use the inhaler while standing up.
3. Open your mouth and place the nozzle of the inhaler about an inch in front of your lips. As you begin to breathe in, squeeze the canister and continue to inhale the spray as long as possible, usually for about two to three seconds.
4. Close your mouth, hold your breath, and count silently to five.
5. When you finally exhale, do so slowly, as if breathing out through a straw.
6. Wait five to ten minutes, then repeat steps 3 through 5.

An aerosolized medication starts working within five to ten minutes after use, and the therapeutic effect can last from four to six hours in most patients. A child may safely use *no more* than two puffs every four to six hours. This equals a maximum of twelve puffs every twenty-four hours. If you feel more is necessary, speak with your physician.

Warning: When *any* MDI is used, be attentive to the way the child handles it and be on the lookout for abuse. If a medicine works well, it is only human nature for parents to haul it out every time their child's condition takes a turn for the worse, even a small turn. In the hands of a youngster who has no real sense of the potential toxicity of a drug, the temptation to use it at will is twice as great, and surreptitious overuse can become a dangerous habit. Many children under twelve years old are not mature enough to handle the responsibility which the self-administration of any strong medicine requires, and it is suggested that parents *never* give a child carte blanche with an inhaler or, for that matter, with a potent medicine of any kind.

As a help in this direction, note that most hand-held aerosolized nebulizers contain approximately 200 sprays. Thus, make it a habit to record the date on which the canister is first put into use, then make note of the day on which it becomes empty. In this way you will be able to monitor how many sprays per day are being taken. If the number is larger than ten (that is, if the medicine is used up within twenty days or less) a serious discussion should take place between the patient, parents and physician.

Bitolterol Marketed as Tornalate in MDI form, bitolterol is the newest of the beta-adrenergic aerosol preparations. The drug is recommended for patients twelve and older; according to its manufacturer, its duration of action is eight hours. I have not been overly impressed with this medication. My patients have complained about its bitter taste, and its period of effective action appears to be less than advertised.

Fenoterol and Procaterol While both these beta-adrenergic drugs are prescribed in many countries around the world, doctors are still awaiting FDA approval for their use in the United States. These drugs will probably be on the market within one to two years.

The role of beta-adrenergic drugs Why use a beta-adrenergic agent when theophylline is in most cases a perfectly adequate antiasthma agent?

Some children cannot tolerate a dose of theophylline large enough to achieve a therapeutic blood level. With the addition of a beta agent to the treatment regimen, asthma symptoms that failed to improve with low doses of theophylline will often respond to a combination of both drugs.

Beta-adrenergic aerosols are especially effective in blocking the development of exercise-induced asthma.

Aerosolized beta-adrenergic preparations can be taken *ahead of time* when parents know that their child is entering an allergy-sensitive environment —for example, when visiting someone who owns animals or when traveling from the city to the country during pollen season. As a case in point, if Ron is allergic to Aunt Tillie's cat and if there is a family function being held at

Table 4. Beta-Adrenergic Bronchodilators

Generic Name	Brand Name	How Administered	Peak Clinical Effect	Duration of Action (in hours)	Common Side Effects and General Comments
Epinephrine					
	Adrenaline solution	By injection	15–20 minutes	½–1	Jitteryness, nausea, vomiting, rapid heartbeat
	Sus-Phrine suspension	By injection	1–3 hours	4–6	Jitteryness, nausea, vomiting, rapid heartbeat
	Primatene Mist	By MDI	15–20 minutes	½	Not recommended for use as an over-the-counter preparation
	Bronkaid Mist	By MDI	15–20 minutes	½	An over-the-counter preparation that is not recommended for use
Isoproterenol					
	Isuprel HCl solution	By nebulizer	5 minutes	1½–2	Side effects similar to those of epinephrine. Some people have an effect opposite to the usual response, which may aggravate the asthma symptoms.
	Isuprel Mistometer	By MDI	5 minutes	1½–2	Same as for Isuprel HCl solution. There are several more effective aerosol preparations currently available.
	Medihaler-Iso	By MDI	5 minutes	1½–2	Same as for Isuprel HCl solution

Table 4. (Continued)

Generic Name	Brand Name	How Administered	Peak Clinical Effect	Duration of Action (in hours)	Common Side Effects and General Comments
Isoetharine					
	Bronkosol solution	By nebulizer	5 minutes	1½–2	Side effects similar to those of epinephrine or isoproterenol, but less severe
	Bronkometer	By MDI	5 minutes	1½–2	Same as for Bronkosol solution
Ephedrine					
		Orally	60 minutes	2–3½	Same as for epinephrine. More effective preparations are currently available.
Metaproterenol sulfate					
	Alupent	Tablet	2–2.5 hours	5	Side effects similar to those of epinephrine or isoproterenol but less severe. Shakiness due to muscle tremor is most annoying effect. Given orally it produces fewer side effects than the other beta agents, but muscle tremor still occurs in some patients.
		Syrup	2–2.5 hours	5	
		MDI	15 minutes	4–6	
	Metaprel	Tablet	2–2.5 hours	5	
		Syrup	2–2.5 hours	5	
		MDI	15 minutes	4–6	

Table 4. (Continued)

Generic Name	Brand Name	How Administered	Peak Clinical Effect	Duration of Action (in hours)	Common Side Effects and General Comments
Albuterol					
	Ventolin	Tablet	2 hours	6–8	Fewer effects than other beta agents but muscle tremor can occur
		Syrup	2 hours	6–8	
		MDI	15 minutes	6–8	
	Proventil	Tablet	2 hours	6–8	
		Syrup	2 hours	6–8	
		MDI	15 minutes	6–8	
Terbutaline sulfate					
	Bricanyl	Tablet	2–4 hours	4–6	When injected, produces side effects similar to those of epinephrine. Tremor possible when given orally or by MDI.
		By injection	30–60 minutes	4–8	
	Brethine	Tablet	2–4 hours	4–6	Same as for Bricanyl
		By injection	30–60 minutes	4–8	
	Brethaire	MDI	15 minutes	6–8	

Table 4. (*Continued*)

Generic Name	Brand Name	How Administered	Peak Clinical Effect	Duration of Action (in hours)	Common Side Effects and General Comments
Bitolterol mesylate					
	Tornalate	By MDI	15 minutes	8	Possibly the longest acting of all available MDI beta-adrenergic agents
Fenoterol					
	Berotec	Orally	2–4 hours	6–8	Not yet approved for use in the United States by the FDA
		By MDI	15 minutes	6–8	

her home, the MDI can be used ten minutes before the party begins. Ron then has a good chance of passing a pleasant afternoon visiting with his relatives rather than spending his day outside the house having an asthma attack.

PREVENTATIVE MEDICATION   *Cromolyn sodium*   The bronchodilator medicines we have discussed so far are all used to control asthma symptoms once they begin. Cromolyn sodium (Intal), on the other hand, has a prophylactic action. This means it can block allergic reactions *before* they begin; it also can decrease to some extent the hyperirritability of the bronchial tree. In my opinion, for most patients who require chronic medication, cromolyn sodium (Intal) should be considered along with theophylline as a first-line treatment for asthma.

As with any medication, Intal will not be effective for all patients. Sticking to a regular dosing schedule will definitely increase the chances that cromolyn will control your child's asthma.

How does it work? As mentioned earlier, asthmatic children have hyperreactivity of the bronchial airways as a basic physiologic abnormality. Cromolyn sodium when taken on a regular basis (four times a day) has the potential to diminish this increased responsiveness. It also blocks the release from the mast cells of histamine and other asthma-causing substances.

An example of this drug in action concerns Jason, whose best friend happened to own a large, friendly calico cat. Whenever Jason walked into his friend's house, he felt entirely normal. Within ten minutes he began to cough and wheeze, and a few minutes after that he was in the midst of a full-fledged asthmatic attack. When it was determined that the animal was causing the trouble, Jason's doctor prescribed Intal and told Jason to take the drug immediately before entering cat territory. Now Jason plays regularly at his friend's house for two to three hours at a time without any discomfort—but only when he remembers to take his medicine beforehand.

When is cromolyn prescribed? An increasing number of allergists today consider cromolyn, along with theophylline and the beta-adrenergic agents, to be a first-line drug, which means that many children do well on it alone and require no further medication. As stated, however, cromolyn is prophylactic: it must be taken *before* an asthma attack has started when the lung passageways are free of obstruction. Once bronchospasms begin and the child is actively wheezing, cromolyn is largely ineffective.

Because it is a prophylactic drug and must be taken three to four times a day in order to be effective, cromolyn should be prescribed only for children who suffer from chronic asthma and who require medication on an ongoing basis. Except in certain specific situations (mentioned below where exercise-induced asthma is discussed), it is by no means a one-time medicine.

Cromolyn must sometimes be taken for several weeks before its full effectiveness becomes apparent. A fair trial is always in order: the child should take one capsule by Spinhaler or two puffs with the MDI four times a day for four to six weeks. If, and only if, there is no clinical improvement whatsoever at the end of this period can you assume that cromolyn is not effective for your child.

Cromolyn is particularly effective in blocking the type of asthma that results from strenuous physical exertion, known as EIA. Taking one capsule by Spinhaler or two puffs of the MDI twenty minutes before recess, gym class or general playtime is an effective way to keep an active child symptom free. When administered immediately before exposure to an allergen such as animal dander, cromolyn can also suppress an allergic response.

How is the drug administered? Cromolyn sodium is currently available in three dosage forms: in a metered-dose inhaler, as a powder (in a capsule) and as a solution (in a glass ampule). The powder is inhaled from a small hand-held device called a Spinhaler. For younger patients who cannot use the spinhaler, the cromolyn sodium solution is used with a small compressed air pump. The air pump converts the cromolyn solution to an aerosol mist that the patient inhales through a face mask.

The mechanics of the spinhaler operation are as follows:

1. The cromolyn sodium (Intal) capsule is placed in the spinhaler.
2. The capsule is punctured by sliding the barrel of the spinhaler down and up.
3. The child places the spinhaler in his mouth and inhales deeply. It may take two to six deep breaths in order to empty the powder from the capsule.

Side effects Extended studies of cromolyn show a very low incidence of harmful side effects, and those which do occur are generally quite mild. The most common symptoms are coughing, a transient wheeze, or a slight sore throat.

The starting dose is one capsule four times a day. This schedule is continued for one month. Those patients who have a good response may be continued on as little as two capsules a day. If your child should wheeze or cough after inhaling cromolyn sodium, this reaction can almost always be blocked by pretreatment with an aerosolized beta-adrenergic bronchodilator. The bronchodilator MDI dose inhaler should be used five minutes before taking Intal. Generally speaking, cromolyn is one of the safest drugs on the asthma and allergy market today.

There is, however, one area in which problems may arise. It is not from the drug itself, ironically, but from the patient, the patient's family and the physician. If the doctor fails to stress the importance of complying with instructions for the use of cromolyn and does not demonstrate the proper handling of the Spinhaler, then the patient is unlikely to make the proper use of the medicine. Why?

The major problem associated with the successful long-term administration of any medication is compliance. Most people just don't like taking medicine, and that is doubly true if you don't feel sick! If Intal is working effectively, your child will have few or no asthma symptoms. It is at this time that you as a parent must be most diligent in making sure that the medicine is taken regularly.

The other concern shared by parents and physicians regarding the use of chronic medication relates to the possible harmful side effects caused by the specific drug. On this point let me reassure you that cromolyn sodium is one of the safest medications I have prescribed in the past twenty years. Studies carried out worldwide confirm my personal observations.

If this medicine is prescribed for your child, I urge you to give it a fair trial before making a decision regarding its effectiveness.

CORTICOSTEROIDS   *General comments* The many steroid preparations available today are all derived from cortisone, a natural hormone produced by the adrenal glands, those cap-shaped, adrenaline-producing organs located atop the kidneys. Steroids have been used for the treatment of severe asthma and other allergic conditions for the past twenty years, and they have undoubtedly saved the lives of many, many children, but they are a double-edged sword. On the one hand, steroids have the ability to relieve a great deal of suffering; on the other, they can cause much misery. The responsibility for steering you through these potentially dangerous waters falls squarely on the physician's shoulders.

What are these dangers? The list of potential side effects caused by cortisone reads like a pathology textbook. They range from trifles such as increased appetite to extremely serious conditions such as limitation of physical growth, increased incidence of fractured bones, cataracts and ulcer formation.

At this point you may be making a vow never to let your child be treated with corticosteroids of any kind, ever. On the basis of what has been said, I can hardly blame you, but I hope that when you read the pages that follow, you will be reassured that if cortisone is prescribed in an appropriate dose and for a short period of time, the chances of serious side effects are extremely small. Indeed, in the overall scheme of asthma therapy, it is absolutely necessary for you to understand when steroids should and should not be used, and to place them in their deserved perspective:

Cortisone and its derivatives should *not* be the first medicine given for an acute asthma attack. When first administered they can take as long as four to eight hours to work, and this is simply too long.

Theophylline and the beta-adrenergic bronchodilators should be the first drugs to be used for an acute asthmatic attack. Only if these medications fail to adequately control symptoms should cortisone be considered.

If a decision has been made to use a cortisone preparation, then it should be administered in the proper dosage and for the shortest period of time needed to do its job, usually less than ten to fourteen days.

If cortisone is to be used for five days or less, there is no reason to taper the dose, i.e., reduce it from five pills a day to four, then to three, etc. For example, a dose of four pills a day can be given for five straight days and then abruptly discontinued.

The dose *should* be tapered if cortisone is to be given for more than a week.

Of the many cortisone derivative preparations commercially available I prefer to use an intermediate-acting form such as prednisone or methyl-prednisolone. These agents have had a somewhat lower incidence of harmful side effects than the longer-acting forms of cortisone such as dexamethasone and betamethasone.

How do they work? Cortisone works in the following ways to help control asthma:

1. Because of its ability to reduce inflammation (anti-inflammatory property), it decreases the irritation and mucous congestion in the bronchial tubes.
2. The lungs respond better to the bronchodilator drugs the patient is taking.
3. There is some evidence but no conclusive proof that steroids relax the bronchial smooth muscle spasms that are a major problem for all children with asthma.

Remember that the clinical effects of cortisone are not apparent until two to eight hours after the medicine has been taken.

How are corticosteroids administered? Cortisone and its derivatives may be administered in tablet form, as a liquid, by injection, as an aerosol spray, or intravenously.

Most commonly, steroids are administered orally, either as a liquid, tablet or aerosol spray. Intravenous methods are generally limited to hospital situations, while injections are rarely necessary and are used only when the doctor suspects that the patient is not taking the medicine as prescribed. Table 5 provides the names of the most commonly used oral forms.

Side effects During the period a child is taking cortisone, parents should be certain that the doctor makes constant efforts to decrease both the dose and the length of time the drug is given. As there is a direct relationship between dose, duration of treatment, and the development of side effects, the possibility of overuse must be meticulously guarded against by everyone involved.

This is an extremely critical point to understand. Cortisone rarely causes

Table 5. *Oral Corticosteroid Preparations*

Generic Name	Brand Name	Available Dosages, in Milligrams	Equivalent Strength,* in Milligrams	Ability to Suppress Adrenal Function	Side Effects†		Duration of action per Single Dose (in hours)
					Increase Appetite	Muscle Pains	
		Short-acting					
Cortisone	Cortisone Acetate tablets	5, 10, 25	25	2+	2+	1+	8–12
Hydrocortisone	Hydrocortisone. Cortef tablets	5, 10, 20	20	2+	2+	1+	8–12
		Intermediate-acting					
Prednisone	Prednisone USP tablets / Deltasone tablets / Meticorten tablets	1, 2, 5, 10, 20, 50	5	2+	3+	1+	12–36
Prednisolone	Prednisolone USP tablets / Delta-Cortef tablets	1, 2.5, 5	5	2+	3+	1+	12–36

Table 5. (Continued)

Generic Name	Brand Name	Available Dosages, in Milligrams	Equivalent Strength,* in Milligrams	Side Effects†			
				Ability to Suppress Adrenal Function	Increase Appetite	Muscle Pains	Duration of action per Single Dose (in hours)
Methylprednisolone	Methylprednisolone (Medrol) tablets	2, 4, 8, 16, 24, 32	4	2+	2+	1+	12–36
Triamcinolone	Triamcinolone tablets	1, 2, 4, 8, 16	4	3+	1+	3+	24–48
	Aristocort tablets	2–4					
	Kenacort liquid	5 cc					
Long-acting							
Dexamethasone	Dexamethasone tablets	0.25, 0.5, 0.75, 1.5, 4.0	0.75	4+	4+	2+	36–54
Betamethasone	Decadron tablets	0.60	0.60	4+	4+	2+	36–54
	Celestone tablets						

*Equivalent strength denotes the dosage amount, in milligrams, necessary to achieve an equal effect.

†Side effect reactions are graded on a scale from 1 to 4+, with 1 being the weakest reaction and 4+ the strongest.

problems when treatment is limited to a 5- to 10-day course. When given for more than two weeks, side effects will probably begin, albeit lesser ones such as increased appetite or weight gain. If daily treatment continues for a month or more, potentially serious adverse effects can and do often occur. These may include:

- a decrease in the function of the adrenal glands
- a slowing of the child's growth rate (If given for long enough in a high enough dose, steroids can induce premature closure of the growth centers in the bones, stopping the child's physical growth *entirely.*)
- a decrease in resistance to infection
- changes in the skin, with a tendency to the development of acne, stretch marks and excess body hair
- adverse effects on the contours of the child's face, producing what is called a "moon facies"—an exaggeratedly rounded or "moon face"
- headaches, insomnia and dizziness
- stomach and intestinal problems, with the possibility of stomach ulcers
- the formation of cataracts
- serious kidney complications
- psychological disturbances such as depression

Unfortunately, this is only a partial list of possible side effects associated with prolonged high doses of this powerful drug. The development of unwanted side effects from corticosteroid drugs is related to the dose of medication, how the medicine is administered and the duration of treatment. The incidence and severity of these harmful side effects can be minimized by regulating the amount of drug administered, the length of time the medication is taken, the dosage form used and the dosing schedule.

Earlier in this section, I stated my preference for using an intermediate-acting steroid such as prednisone or prednisolone over the longer-acting forms like betamethasone and dexamethasone. Medical researchers have shown that forms of cortisone which are rapidly metabolized (used up) by the body are less likely to cause injury to the adrenal glands. These glands are the source of cortisone in the body and are essential for life.

Longer-acting forms of cortisone such as betamethasone and dexamethasone exert their effects on the body two or three times longer than either prednisone and prednisolone. Therefore, these long-acting drugs have a greater tendency to suppress adrenal gland function.

When prescribing a cortisone preparation, I try to use the smallest dose for the shortest period that will produce the desired clinical response. The goal should always be to discontinue cortisone as soon as possible.

If steroids are used for four- to seven-day periods and then stopped, the possibility that any long-lasting side effects will develop is extremely small.

With the exception of a patient who had an increase in appetite, I cannot recall seeing anyone who has had a significant problem with a short course of cortisone.

If it becomes necessary to keep a child on longer-term cortisone therapy because of severe asthma, then the methods of choice are the use of an aerosolized preparation given three to four times a day or the oral administration of a preparation such as prednisone given as a single dose once every other morning. This is known as an alternate-day schedule. Using either of these techniques significantly reduces the incidence of harmful side effects. You should discuss these options with your child's doctor.

Monitoring steroids As yet, there is no practical way to monitor steroid levels in the blood in the way that we can monitor theophylline. If a child must use high doses of cortisone for prolonged periods of time, periodic checks of adrenal gland function may be necessary. A variety of blood tests can be used to determine whether there is any impairment of adrenal function. The need for such tests arises infrequently, and then only for children who have been on cortisone for extended periods of time.

Summary of suggestions and recommendations for the use of steroids Steroids are such potent drugs that a review of the caveats issued so far is in order. Here are your major concerns if your child's asthma is serious enough to warrant steroid treatment.

Make sure your doctor uses steroids only when they are absolutely necessary; that is, only when all other asthma drugs have been tried and have not provided adequate relief. This is the first and the last rule of steroid administration. If steroids are required, make sure that the smallest necessary dose is used for the shortest possible period of time.

I prefer to see a child receive his total twenty-four-hour dose of steroids as a single morning dose. After medication is given for a four- to seven-day course, it may then be discontinued. If cortisone is needed for more than ten to fourteen days, the dose should be gradually decreased for a period of time before being discontinued.

If it becomes necessary to give repeated short pulse doses of cortisone over a three-to-six-month period, your doctor should recommend the alternate-day method of treatment. If your child is old enough to use a metered dose inhaler, an aerosolized steroid preparation is probably the safest method of administration.

Any child who has taken cortisone for a month or more will almost certainly develop some degree of adrenal gland suppression. While this condition is reversible, it may take as long as a year before adrenal gland function returns to normal. During this period, if particularly stressful circumstances occur—such as a severe infection or the need for surgery

—it may be necessary to give cortisone for several days until the acute episode has passed. This procedure, to repeat, is required only for children who have used corticosteroids for long periods of time.

If the long-term use of a corticosteroid is absolutely necessary, it is the doctor's responsibility to discuss with the parents the risks involved *before* these medications are administered. Any doctor who prescribes large doses of steroids for extended periods of time without first talking it over with the family is, in my opinion, practicing bad medicine.

Long-term oral steroids should be given in the lowest possible effective dose. Every effort must be made on the physician's part to constantly lower and ultimately discontinue their use.

Steroids should be the last drug used in the treatment of chronic asthma and the first one discontinued. If your child is given steroids before first being tried on theophylline, the beta-adrenergics and cromolyn, something is wrong. Find out what it is. Perhaps a second opinion is in order. At least bring the subject to light with your doctor and ask why he is using these potent medications. If the answer does not satisfy you, and if a second opinion justifies your doubt, consider switching physicians.

ANTIBIOTICS   Most children who wheeze in association with an upper respiratory tract infection will *not* benefit from the use of antibiotics. The reason is simple: most colds are caused by viruses, not by bacteria. Currently available antibiotics do not kill viruses, so to prescribe an antibiotic for a viral infection will accomplish very little. The only time antibiotics really earn their keep is when a serious bacterial infection such as a strep throat or ear infection is associated with the asthma. Then such a drug is clearly in order. If some question arises as to whether or not an infection is viral or bacterial, a visit to the doctor for advice is the best move.

Using antibiotics for asthma and allergies   Erythromycin, an antibiotic frequently prescribed for children, may cause problems for any asthmatic youngster who is also taking theophylline. The antibiotic slows down the metabolism of theophylline, which can lead to an increased level of theophylline in the blood. In this situation, signs and symptoms of theophylline toxicity may develop. I would advise you to become familiar with these symptoms as described on page 71 and to be on the watch for them.

Questions have been raised regarding the use of penicillin for an allergic child with asthma. Currently, there is no evidence to indicate that an allergic child runs a greater risk of developing an allergic penicillin reaction than a nonallergic, nonasthmatic child.

Finally, let me repeat that under most circumstances an asthma attack will *not* require the use of antibiotics as part of the usual course of treatment. When a bacterial infection is associated with acute asthma symptoms, then treatment with these drugs is absolutely necessary. Unfortunately, most child-hood infections, especially those involving the upper respiratory tract, are caused by viruses, against which antibiotics are of no assistance. It has been my experience that only a relatively small percentage of children with acute asthma really require an antibiotic.

EXPECTORANTS   One of the major problems that children have during an asthma attack is the accumulation of large amounts of thick, sticky mucus in the lungs. Expectorants are supposed to thin these secretions and make them easier to eliminate.

In theory this sounds great, but to date the pharmaceutical companies have been unable to produce any expectorants that are really effective. Indeed, if the truth be told, the best expectorant is plain old H_2O, though fluids in any form, hot or cold, are as effective as the commercial products you purchase at the drugstore.

Among the available expectorant preparations, probably the most com-monly prescribed are those containing guaifenesin. Some well-known examples include the Robitussin family of cough preparations, the many forms of Nalde-con and over sixty others as listed in the 1986 *Physicians' Desk Reference.* Iodides have been used as expectorants for a long time, but many teenagers cannot tolerate these preparations because of their side effects. Some of these include: acne-like skin eruptions, nausea, vomiting and possible development of an enlarged thyroid.

To summarize: while there are a number of expectorant preparations on the market today, none are highly effective. My first choice for an expectorant is simply plenty of palatable liquids, in whatever form your child will accept and as much as he will swallow. In the long run, water is best of all.

ANTIHISTAMINES   For children unlucky enough to have both asthma and allergic rhinitis there exists a lot of confusion regarding the use of antihista-mines. The theoretical reason for not prescribing antihistamines is their po-tential to dry out the mucus in the bronchial tubes, which would worsen asthma symptoms. In practice this problem rarely occurs. In my experience, if a child is regularly taking a bronchodilator I cannot recall any situation when asthma symptoms increased after an antihistamine was taken. Re-cently, some evidence has been published suggesting that in some patients asthma symptoms have improved while on antihistamines. Although many antihistamines are now available without prescription, I would urge you to discuss your child's specific situation with your allergist or pediatrician be-fore administering these drugs.

Immunotherapy

General comments Most children with asthma do not demonstrate a clear-cut relationship between their attacks and contact with a specific allergen. The child who wheezes *only* during a particular pollen season or who has difficulty breathing *only* when playing with cats or dogs is unusual. When and if such a relationship between asthma sysmptoms and allergen exposure can be definitely established, then—and then only—immunotherapy can be of potential benefit.

Briefly summarized, immunotherapy is a process in which patients are injected with specific allergens to which they have proven to be allergic. Initially, the treatment schedule calls for the injection of highly dilute allergens; gradually the concentration is increased until the patient receives a potent maintenance dose.

An immunotherapy program begins with weekly visits to the doctor. As treatment progresses, the time between visits gradually increases to the point where appointments are required only once a month. The objective of immunotherapy is to produce a level of immunity to a specific allergen so that patients will no longer develop asthma symptoms when exposed to the specific substance(s).

Managing the Child with Chronic Asthma

Asthmatic Children and Family Trauma: Don't Underestimate the Strain

Because of the time, effort and expense required to care for a child with chronic asthma, the stress parents suffer can become as severe as the child's symptoms. In my own practice I have seen marriages break up due to the pressures an asthmatic child's needs and demands exert on parents. These stresses filter down through the entire family structure, disrupting life on many levels, making the simplest things difficult in a thousand ways.

For example, a long-time family pet must suddenly be given away to friends; the best explanation the parents can come up with to rationalize this seemingly cruel act is that the animal "makes Tommy wheeze." "So what!" cry Tommy's brothers and sisters, and rebellion fills the air. Meanwhile, Tommy's food sensitivities turn daily kitchen activities into an uphill battle, forcing Mother to prepare two separate meals, one for her asthmatic child, one for everyone else. Beloved family activities are curtailed or even ended completely: camping, antique-hunting, picnicking, touch football games, dining out, visits to the zoo—all go by the boards. Parents in turn become tyrannical over what were once petty concerns, screaming at their children lest they track asthma-causing dust into the house or forget to close a window. Special attentions are lavished on Tommy while the needs of the other brothers and sisters —in their minds, at any rate—are neglected. On and on it goes, the pressures increasing as the asthma drags on, parents, siblings and sick child lining up one against the other in endless confrontations, all of which, it somehow seems, end up centered around poor Tommy's "condition."

What's the remedy? I have no cure-alls for you, but some things will definitely help.

Talking frankly about Tommy's asthma with all family members is a good starting point. Acknowledge that problems *do* exist and that everyone in the family has a part to play in eliminating them or at least reducing them. Pretending, wearing rose-colored glasses to protect the sick child and other family members, making believe that everything is just fine and that Tommy's difficulties are "just a phase" will only make matters worse.

Agree to work together *as a family team* to make things better, both for the patient and for the entire family.

Begin by looking for alternatives to activities that the child's asthma has made impractical. If the seashore is out for vacations, try the mountains or the desert or a cabin by a lake or even a summer visit to an interesting city. If it's no longer feasible to fill your house with overstuffed antique chairs, start collecting contemporary furnishings instead. In other words, instead of nursing antagonisms over lost pleasures, be creative. Think of ways to replace them.

When an especially heavy load falls on a single family member, help out. Divide the labor and let everyone pitch in. If extra housecleaning is required to keep the dust down, if special meals must be prepared, make sure that everyone does his or her share. Such combined efforts will not only lighten everyone's labor but will provide that special satisfaction which comes from working together as a mutually caring team.

Don't be afraid to seek professional counseling if you feel you and your family need it. If pressures in an asthmatic household become too great, a visit to a therapist or family counselor may be just what is needed. These professionals are specially trained to help in stressful situations, and you may be surprised to hear the interesting, timely and unexpected suggestions they come up with. By no means should you take such a visit as an admission of failure or as a sign that you or the child are "sick." Nor should you suppose that by visiting a counselor you are roping yourself into years and years on the couch. Often, after a few open and pertinent counseling sessions, families have received all the help they need. From then on, problems that previously seemed insurmountable are handled with relative ease.

Self-Management Techniques for the Asthmatic Child: How Does It Work?

The more an asthmatic child is encouraged to manage his own condition, the better off everyone will be, including the child. By self-management I do *not* mean that your child should serve as his own doctor. Of course not. Self-management means that both the parents and the child gather as much information as possible concerning what can safely be done at home to help the asthma, and that they put this information into practice, regularly and systematically, without fail.

First, talk with your doctor. Get the hard facts and integrate them into your approach to your child's day-to-day welfare. Find out:

- what your child can safely do at home to manage the condition
- how you as a parent can help
- how you can learn to gauge when a situation is self-manageable and when it is not
- how to know when to call the doctor for advice

Any responsible physician will be willing to spend time with you on these details and provide the information necessary to start a program of successful self-management. Before you begin, make sure you are clear on all the details.

Ask questions. If you don't understand something the doctor said concerning self-management, say so. Be certain you get it all. If you are unsure why you must give your child a particular medicine every six hours or what the reason is for taking an aerosol treatment every morning, you will probably not be very effective in making sure that the job gets done. On the other hand, if you know why certain procedures must be carried out at certain times and in certain ways, you will be far more likely to follow instructions. So ask. Don't be satisfied until you feel confident in your knowledge.

Once you have a course of self-management set up, comply with it carefully. One possible reason asthma attacks continue to occur among children who are under a doctor's care is that both the parents and patient do not carefully comply with the doctor's recommendations. In other words, failure to follow the daily medicine routine will inevitably encourage the development of symptoms. Common sense tells us this must be so. And while there is no guarantee that sticking to a set course of medication will always prevent such episodes from occurring, certainly *failing* to follow medical instructions is quite likely to lead to an attack.

The Active Asthmatic Child: How to Go About Regulating an Asthmatic Child's Activities

In my experience, some parents tend to overprotect asthmatic children from many types of stressful activities, mental or physical, out of fear that these situations will trigger an attack. The children of such parents may eventually find themselves deprived of childhood's most essential pleasures: sports, trips to the beach, games, visits to the country, pillow fights, eating out, keeping pets, spending the night at the home of a buddy. Sometimes these children are overprotected into a state of passivity or helplessness. In dealing with chronic asthma you must establish a set of guidelines appropriate to the child's particular limitations. But isn't it better that these guidelines emphasize freedoms rather than limitations? Better to think in terms of possible dos than in absolute don'ts?

To begin, everyone—physician, patient and parents—should discuss *together* the limits to be placed on a child's activities. Guidelines reached through a consensus are more likely to be followed than those handed down, as it were, from above by an overbearing physician or a set of inflexible parents.

These guidelines can be agreed upon in the doctor's office when everybody is present. Everyone should have a say in the matter of which sports Johnny or Susie can participate in, what toys they can or cannot keep in their room, what pets are safe to have in the house. When deciding these questions, keep one especially important rule in mind: *Base decisions on actual asthma experiences, not theoretical possibilities.* Because Jonathan wheezes whenever he visits a farm is no reason to suppose that young Elisabeth will do the same. Until you know for certain that Elisabeth's asthma is triggered by barnyard animals, visits to farms should be allowed.

In other words, avoid comparing your child to other asthmatic children. Each case is different, each has its own problems, each requires a separate medical strategy. Try not to generalize. The boundaries set on a child's comings and goings depend to a large extent on age, severity of asthma, and the child's ability to accept directions responsibly. The guiding factor behind it all should be allowing the most freedom possible and forbidding an activity *only* when it is proven to trigger an attack. The goal in setting limits is to work toward fewer and fewer restrictions, not toward more and more.

Added to these goals should be an effort to prevent asthmatic children from feeling that they are somehow being punished by the restrictions placed on them, or that the various no's and don'ts invoked for their protection are necessarily permanent. Children's minds, especially younger children's minds, work differently from those of adults. Even if their pleasures are eliminated in the high-sounding name of good health or everyone's "best interests," most will automatically assume they have done something wrong to deserve this deprivation. When they are forced to comply with these limitations, they will feel that they are being disciplined. Make clear to the child that these measures are being taken to protect, not to punish, and that they will change and be modified as the condition itself changes. However you choose to handle this delicate situation, make it a rule never to let a child believe that the curtailment of favorite activities is either permanent or punitive.

Preparing in Advance for an Asthmatic Attack

Here it is, plain and simple: There is absolutely no doubt that the way in which parents deal with their child's asthma can have a significant effect on the severity of the attack. If a parent becomes hysterical whenever his child starts to wheeze, if the household suddenly becomes filled with excited shrieks about hospitals and oxygen masks, if a mad search ensues for the MDI and the medicine bottle, then the child will invariably pick up on the frenzy and her asthma will become accordingly intense. It simply works that way. During a severe asthmatic episode the child will look to you for strength, clear instructions and a sense of calmness. It's up to you to provide all three.

Prepare yourself for the situation ahead of time.

Learn the early warning signs of asthma. As soon as they appear, take the appropriate medical steps immediately. Do not wait until the attack has time to develop before giving medication. For children who have rapid onset of severe symptoms, the wearing of a Medic Alert bracelet may be appropriate in case attacks occur away from home. Have a clear plan for handling an attack. Discuss it with your doctor so that you have confidence in your ability to handle the situation.

Keep all necessary medications, aerosol pumps, instructions, prescriptions, lists, notes, records, phone numbers (including those for the doctor, hospital and ambulance corps) and books pertaining to your child's asthma in a well-marked, accessible location. Running around at the onset of an attack looking for these things will only add to the confusion. Get organized ahead of time and stay that way.

With careful observation, discover everything you can about the patterns and eccentricities of your child's asthma. Learn to identify the signs and symptoms of a mild asthma attack versus an asthma emergency. The more you learn and understand in this regard, the more confident you will feel next time an attack begins.

During a severe episode parents must make every effort to appear calm, confident and self-assured. Even if the attack reaches emergency proportions, panicky behavior by the parents will only produce anxiety on the part of the child. At such times parents must be decisive and act with confidence, even if they are uncertain and highly anxious.

Along these lines, a bit of mental preparation may help. Pick a time when all is calm. Sit quietly and systematically think out in advance all the steps you would take should your child have a severe attack. Go over each of these steps one by one: where the medicine is kept, how to measure the dosages, what physical signs to look for, how to get to the hospital emergency room should a trip be necessary, and so forth. Mentally rehearse this process from beginning to end, and as you do, visualize yourself moving through it all with strength and confidence. Assuming that you practice this bit of preparatory thinking at regular intervals, it will help you to be more mentally *and* emotionally in control next time an attack arrives. Stressful situations *can* be prepared for in advance.

Call for medical assistance if you are uncertain as to how to proceed when an attack begins. It is good to try and determine what direction the episode is taking. If it continues to worsen after medication is given, if breathing becomes increasingly labored, if there is a decrease in the child's ability to talk or walk, and if the danger symptoms mentioned on page 60 start to appear, then and only then are emergency tactics appropriate. Again, *knowledge* of the way your child's asthma symptoms progress is crucial.

When Your Child Must Go to the Hospital

Unfortunately, despite our best efforts, many children each year are admitted to hospitals for the treatment of asthma which has become so severe that all outpatient treatments have failed to control the symptoms. These children are in status asthmaticus and require immediate hospitalization. At Babies' Hospital, the children's division of Columbia Presbyterian Medical Center in New York City, status asthmaticus has been *the* most frequent nonsurgical reason for hospitalization. Between four and five hundred children a year are admitted for asthma treatment, and about 1 to 2 percent of these patients are so sick that they must be cared for in the intensive care unit.

Being admitted to a hospital is an unsettling experience, to say the least. Both patient and parent may already be exhausted from sleepless nights, and both will be enervated from the ordeal of the attack, which by now has gone on for many hours or even several days. Upon arriving at the hospital, instead of receiving a respite from this turmoil they will be greeted by the rush-rush atmosphere of the emergency room and the hurry-up-and-wait protocol at the admissions desk.

While there is not a great deal that can be done to make this encounter more pleasant, you can get through the admissions procedure a bit more quickly, as well as help the attending physician get a clearer picture of your child's problem, if you come prepared to answer the following questions related to the attack.

When did the attack begin?
Was there evidence of an accompanying cold or infection?
Was there a fever?
Has there been vomiting or diarrhea since the attack began?
Has your child been drinking fluids? Approximately how much fluid has he or she taken within the past twenty-four hours?
Exactly what medicines has the child taken and in what specific dose? At what time of day and night were they administered?

In the emergency room a variety of medications may be given in an attempt to stop the attack. Which drugs are used depends on how long the episode has been in progress and the type of medications administered at home. The following drugs and procedures are frequently ordered in an emergency room situation.

Adrenalin or epinephrine This is given by injection, most often in the arm. It may be necessary to administer two or three repeated doses at fifteen- to thirty-minute intervals.

Sus-Phrine A long-lasting form of epinephrine. If there has been a good response to Adrenalin in the emergency room, Sus-Phrine is generally given before the child is discharged from the hospital. Its bronchodilator effects usually last from three to six hours.

Aerosolized bronchodilators Such drugs as metaproterenol or isoetharine are mixed with salt water (saline solution) and inhaled through a face mask or through a pipe-shaped mouthpiece. With each breath some of the medication is drawn directly into the lungs. Treatments last from ten to twenty minutes.

IV If none of the preceding measures stops the attack, the doctor may start an intravenous infusion, commonly known as an IV, in order to administer aminophylline, a form of theophylline, and to get more fluids directly into the child's system. The needle on the IV will be inserted into the hand, foot, or in the inside part of the arm opposite the elbow. If your child has already been taking theophylline, a blood test will also be done to determine the theophylline level in the blood. This information will help the doctor to decide on the amount of theophylline to place in the IV.

ABG determination When an attack has been in progress for many hours, significant metabolic changes take place that affect the oxygen content of the blood, the carbon dioxide level, and the relationship between the body's acid and base levels. The doctor can determine if any dangerous imbalances have resulted from these changes by checking the arterial blood gases. This test requires that a blood specimen be taken from an artery and that the specimen be analyzed for its oxygen content, carbon dioxide level, and acidity. Most children admitted to a hospital for asthma will require at least one ABG study and perhaps more, depending on the severity of the attack.

Chest X-ray X-rays may be used to check for the presence of infection— for example, pneumonia—or to locate areas of the lungs that have become blocked or partially collapsed (atelectasis) due to the presence of mucus plugs. In a very small number of cases, X-ray studies will also be ordered to determine if, due to the popping of a small air sac during an especially severe attack, air has escaped from the lungs and entered the chest cavity, a condition known as pneumomediastinum. In some cases escaped air will also penetrate into the thorax region resulting in a condition called pneumothorax; the heart area, causing pneumopericardium; or the subcutaneous tissues of the upper chest and neck regions, causing subcutaneous emphysema. The diagnosis of this last condition can be made by running the fingers along the chest and neck of the patient; the presence of free air within the tissues will produce a sound similar to that of crinkling cellophane. This condition, though bizarre, usually disappears without medical assistance. More serious are pneumothorax and pneumopericardium, both of which may cause serious compression of the lungs and the heart and are thus potentially life-threatening. Observation and treatment in an intensive care unit are required if these problems develop.

Corticosteroids Once the decision has been made to admit your child to a hospital, the preceding treatments will be given on a continuous basis. If there are no signs of improvement after a six- or twelve-hour period, your doctor may then begin a short course of steroids. Initially these drugs are given through an IV for several days. After this period of time the vast majority of children are well enough to take their medicine by mouth and are soon ready to be discharged from the hospital.

As indicated, hospitalization can be a traumatic experience both for the parents and the child. One way of reducing the shock is by asking questions whenever a procedure takes place that you do not understand. We all become less fearful when we know why particular things are being done to us or to our loved ones. It is your right to have this knowledge. It is your duty to ask these questions.

A Few Additional Thoughts for the Asthmatic Child

Keep your child's weight under control. An overweight condition and asthma are a bad combination for several important reasons. If your child is overweight, the excess poundage will affect his already strained ability to remain lively and to participate in games and sports. Asthma tends to make some children passive wallflowers, especially those who are pampered by their parents and of whom nothing is asked or expected. Excess weight will compound the problem.

Being overweight places an additional strain on the heart. Owing to the increased workload placed on a youngster's cardiac system during an asthmatic episode, fatigue will develop quickly and the child will have less available energy to cope with the attack.

A patient's extra weight makes it particularly difficult for the doctor to calculate appropriate doses of asthma medications.

As most parents will agree, asthmatic youngsters often think of themselves as being different from other children. Add to this already unhealthy situation the negative body image that excess weight invariably produces and you have a double jeopardy. Whenever possible, make sure your child keeps her weight under control. Why add further problems to an already complicated situation?

Physical activity is important. This point is so important that I'll say it again: asthmatic children should be encouraged to participate in a regular program of sports, games and age-appropriate play. I would rather see an asthmatic child take constant medication and, as a result, actively engage in athletics than take no medicine at all and stand sulkily behind the playground fence like an outcast, watching his friends have fun.

Take all the proper commonsense precautions. There are many of these, some obvious, some not. If you smoke, don't do it around your child. Make sure your child gets plenty of fresh, wholesome foods, and eliminate foods you suspect may trigger attacks. When pets cause trouble, squarely face that fact and decide whether or not to place the pet elsewhere, keep it outside, or isolate it in a separate part of the house. Make sure that all responsible members of the family know how to help out with medication schedules and self-treatment methods, and be sure others are carefully trained to do this work should you for whatever reason be absent. Avoid planning vacations in areas where you *know* the child will have trouble. Don't leave medicines where they can accidentally fall into the wrong hands, and, of course, keep them away from small children at all times. Make sure you always have a generous supply of necessary medications on hand; don't wait to run out before refilling prescriptions. This is especially true when you are going away on vacation. Make sure you have an adequate supply of medicine. Alert all teachers in school concerning your child's condition and seek their cooperation. Keep the home environment as stable and serene as possible, and don't forget the value of a sense of humor in coping with just about *any* problem. See to it that the child understands his or her asthma, how it works, what it is, why it occurs, what to expect; the more informed a child is on this subject, the less fearful she is likely to be in time of attack.

Learn all you can about the disease. The more knowledgeable every family member is regarding asthma, the more effectively the problem can be managed. Information concerning medications, how to give them, when to take them, usual and unusual side effects and so forth should be acquired, along with a general understanding of what causes asthma.

Your primary information resource is of course your physician. After taking what you can from this source, go to the library, where you'll find many books on allergies and asthma. A national organization with branches in many states, The Asthma and Allergy Foundation of America, produces a variety of informational pamphlets. Local offices of the American Thoracic Society, and in Washington, D.C., the National Institute of Allergy and Infectious Diseases, can be called upon to answer questions and to supply you with a wide selection of educational materials. Take advantage of them. Their addresses are furnished in the Appendix.

Questions and Answers about Asthma

Must an asthmatic child take medicine even when there are no obvious signs of wheezing or shortness of breath?

It depends on the child's particular condition. Bronchodilator drugs, discussed earlier in this chapter, should be taken for at least four to six days after all obvious symptoms of acute asthma have disappeared. Continuing the medicine will permit the patient's lungs to return to a more normal functional level. After this period of time, assuming that all the youngster's symptoms have disappeared, these drugs can be discontinued. If, on the other hand, a child's attacks occur at such frequent intervals that she is never comfortable for more than two or three days at a time, then this child is clearly a chronic sufferer. In such a case I would recommend the use of bronchodilators on a daily schedule.

How exactly do you define "chronic" asthma?

There is probably no single definition agreed on by all physicians. I feel that if a child has undergone repeated attacks of asthma for longer than one year, his case can be described as chronic. At the same time, there is, as in most things, also a matter of degree in any chronic condition, and this may be determined by looking at several revealing variables:

How frequent are the attacks?
How prolonged are the attacks?
How severe are the attacks?
Are the attacks becoming more intense or less intense?
Are the attacks becoming more common or less common?

For example, any child who wheezes several times a week for a period of six months to a year can certainly be said to have chronic asthma. But you might also look at a child who has wheezed only two or three times a year over the past four or five years and also say that, technically, this case is chronic. The two situations are clearly quite different, and I would manage each in an entirely different way: medication on a regular basis for the first situation, medication only during those periods when the child becomes symptomatic in the second. Yet both are technically chronic.

How should an asthmatic child be prepared before undergoing elective surgery?

With our present knowledge and the antiasthma medications available, the potential problems that surgery may entail can be avoided.

Your child should be examined by his or her regular doctor in the week prior to the scheduled operation. At that time a decision will be made regarding which medication, if any, has to be prescribed. If the child's lungs are not completely clear, then a three- to five-day course of prednisone (cortisone) in addition to an oral bronchodilator should be given. If any cortisone preparation has been taken within six months of the surgery date, it is advisable for your child to have a short (three- to five-day) course of an appropriate short-acting steroid.

At the time of the operation, the anesthesiologist, who will be aware of your child's asthma history, will use the anesthetic agent least likely to aggravate or trigger asthma symptoms.

After the surgery, special attention will be given to your child to prevent the development of an asthma attack. These steps may include the use of intravenous aminophylline, an aerosolized bronchodilator, and possibly steroids. The child will be encouraged to do some simple breathing exercises and to cough regularly in order to prevent the accumulation of large amounts of mucus in the lungs.

Today, if your child needs some type of surgery, the fact that he or she has asthma is rarely reason for added concern.

What is the ideal geographic environment for an asthmatic child? What parts of the country are best for this condition?

There is no ideal environment for a person with asthma just as there is no typical asthmatic child. As to safe and unsafe parts of the country, whenever consideration of a move from one geographic area to another is contemplated, there is no way of predicting how such a move will affect the child. Most short-term changes of residence do prove beneficial, but usually only in the beginning. Problems come later on, six months or a year after the move is made. Often the family of a child with respiratory problems will pull up stakes and resettle in a supposedly asthma-free environment such as Arizona. For a while everything is fine; the child's breathing is perfect. Before too long, though, the local pollens, the local air pollution, the local animals, the local allergens all take their toll, and things may be back where they started. Moving solely to escape an allergy is a risky business at best and has no proven medical benefits.

What role does air pollution play in asthma?

There is no question that air pollution of any type—whether from auto emissions, industrial contamination or unusual weather patterns—can have a harmful effect on most asthmatics. The irritating effects on the lungs of various chemical compounds such as sulfur dioxide and carbon monoxide have been responsible for triggering many acute attacks. At best, these chemical irritants aggravate preexisting asthma conditions; in a small but identifiable percentage of patients they may be the cause of the asthma. There are specific indoor-work-related situations in which employees who have been chronically exposed to excessive levels of toxic chemicals develop symptoms of asthma. Some preliminary information suggests that in homes equipped with gas ovens and cooking ranges children with asthma tend to have more symptoms. This early observation is being evaluated in a number of current research projects. In short, both indoor and outdoor air pollution can and in many instances does play a definable role.

Is it ever necessary or advisable to send a child to an asthma residential treatment center?

Fortunately, only a small percentage of childhood asthmatics are so handicapped by their ailment that their school life, social life and family life suffer severe disruptions. Those who are in this category seem to spend most of their time in the doctor's office, emergency room or the hospital being admitted in status asthmaticus. For the benefit of these youngsters and for their families, it may be advisable to consider admitting them to a residential asthma treatment center; a list of these facilities appears in the Appendix.

Residential treatment centers are set up to provide children whose chronic asthma is uncontrollable at home with a period of time away during which they can be taught by professionals how to better cope with their ailment. The staff of these centers is composed of physicians, psychologists, nurses, social workers, schoolteachers, psychotherapists and dietitians, all of whom contribute to a total treatment program tailor-made to the needs of each patient. Children usually remain at these centers from six to twenty-four months.

As a general rule, it is best, if feasible, to find a residential treatment center as close to home as possible. Admitting a child in a center an hour or so from home is less likely to provoke anxiety than shipping him off to an institution fifteen hundred miles away. By using a nearby facility the family can become involved in the educational and treatment program; this is vitally important. An older concept, originally formulated by the physicians who first began the residential centers in Arizona and Denver, of "parentectomy," whereby the child is intentionally separated from the parents to avoid all internal family conflict, has today been repudiated by almost all authorities. Most professionals now feel that the family *must* become intimately involved in the total asthma treatment program if success is to be attained. In fact, educating both parents and child is the major goal of treatment teams at these centers, their basic philosophy being that the more everyone understands about asthma, the more effective everyone will be at coping with it.

Does cigarette smoke bother asthma?

Absolutely and unquestionably. Tobacco smoke is a primary irritant for *anyone* with asthma. It is harmful just to be in a room where cigarette smoke is hanging in the air. As for adolescent asthmatics who take up the cigarette habit, all any doctor can say to them is this: PLEASE STOP NOW! RIGHT NOW! before any real damage is done and before the addiction becomes permanent.

Is there any proof that asthmatic children suffer from emotional problems more frequently than nonasthmatic children?

From my own experience and from most of the evidence we have today, there seem to be no identifiable psychological differences between children with asthma and children without. Among youthful asthma sufferers you will find all personality types, all physical types, all psychological types, all social types —there is no "typical" asthmatic child. Many people have claimed that asthmatic children are loners, preferring their own company to that of others; or that such children are introverted, brooding, even emotionally unstable. I think that children who suffer from any chronic medical problem that keeps them socially isolated from other children and singles them out as strange or different will invariably become a bit withdrawn. In other words, I do not believe it is the personality of the child that contributes to the asthma, but the condition of being asthmatic that affects the personality. Proof of this in my own practice has come from observing the occasional withdrawn child with chronic severe asthma become an outgoing, actively participating member of his social group as his condition is brought under control.

At one time many professionals claimed that "smother love"—i.e., an overbearing, overprotective and overcontrolling attitude on the part of the mother—was a major contributing factor in the development of asthma. Is this theory still given credence?

The whole question of the psychological relationship of the parents to the child, and specifically the mother to the child, vis-à-vis the development of asthma, is an issue that has simply never been settled one way or the other. Some years ago, in an attempt to establish a definite link between asthma and the emotions, psychologists and psychiatrists developed a psychological type they called the asthmatic personality. One of the identifying traits of this type was a domineering mother. The concept has not stood the test of time, and the final verdict is that evidence for its support is inconclusive at best.

There are special summer camps for asthmatic children. How do they differ from regular camps?

In camps established specifically for children with asthma, the counselors and the medical staff are specially trained to deal with asthma-related problems. This means that recreational programs feature less intensely competitive physical activities and that extremely taxing sports such as soccer or distance running are generally avoided. Such camps have both the medical staff and specialized medical facilities equipped to treat the child who develops an acute asthma attack. By and large, however, the sports, games, activities and recreations at a camp oriented to the needs of asthmatic children are not unlike those you might see at a regular camp.

I do not think it is wise to send children to special camps unless they have such severe asthma that they would otherwise not be able to enjoy a summer of active fun. Singling out a youngster and sending him to "special" places may reinforce that child's already developed sense of being sick, of being out of step and strange. Most children with asthma can function quite well at regular camps *provided* they go equipped with proper medication. At least try these camps first and see how things work out.

Do you recommend the use of relaxation techniques such as biofeedback, meditation, hypnosis or autohypnosis for help with asthma?

Any relaxation technique that can help to relieve the anxiety and emotional stress associated with an asthma attack is worth trying. I have been impressed with the lessening of symptoms some patients have exhibited with the use of biofeedback and self-hypnosis. Providing that the patient receives proper instruction from a qualified professional I have no objection to a trial with these techniques. Breathing exercises can be useful techniques for relaxation.

Chronic Rhinitis

Christopher, age nine, is in good health and is a perfectly normal, happy youngster except for a single recurring problem: each year in early spring he begins to sneeze, has a constantly runny nose, and complains of itchy eyes and throat. Like clockwork, these bothersome symptoms start up sometime in April and continue without a break through early July.

Janet, age thirteen, has had a two-year history of nasal congestion. Her problem surfaces in late October when the forced-air heating in her home is turned on and it continues until early spring. Her father is pondering the unpleasant prospect of replacing the entire household heating system.

Angela, age five, has been in nursery school since she was three. There she experiences what appears to be a constant cold with drippy nose, cough and violent sneezing. These symptoms start in September when school begins and continue throughout the school year. Angela's teachers sometimes send her home for fear that other children in the class will catch her "cold," but her parents know better. She, like the others, is a victim of chronic rhinitis.

These three youngsters are representative of a veritable army of children who suffer from a wide range of symptoms, all of which are lumped under a single heading: chronic rhinitis, or as a variety of it is known, hay fever. This maddening disorder affects approximately 20 million Americans each year. In 1975, American children experienced 28 million restricted activity days, 6 million bedridden days, and 2 million days missed from school all due to some form of rhinitis. That same year the national expenditure for hay fever drugs and medical costs exceeded $500 million; the figure has almost doubled since then. While clearly not a life-threatening disorder, rhinitis is responsible for significant personal and economic hardships. It is not, as the worn joke reminds us, something to be sneezed at.

Inside the Nasal Labyrinth

Before details on the different forms of rhinitis that may plague your child are provided, some background on the workings of the nose are in order. Several

111

facts are, of course, obvious. We breathe through our nose, and our sense of smell is located in our nose. It is, however, not entirely accurate to say that this organ serves simply as a breathing tube or as a conduit for odors. In reality, our nose "processes" air as well as draws it in. It filters the air, humidifies it, and regulates its temperature. If these functions are not performed properly we become quite uncomfortable. Sometimes we get downright sick.

Major landmarks to become familiar with here are the three turbinates, extending from the nostrils to the nasopharynx located at the back of the throat (see below). There is an *inferior* turbinate, a *middle* turbinate and a *superior* turbinate.

Look below the inferior turbinate. Here you will see the opening of the passageway connecting the nose with the eye, the nasolacrimal duct. Near it is the middle turbinate which covers the entrances to the frontal, anterior ethmoid and maxillary sinuses, while beneath the superior turbinate you will find the opening to the posterior ethmoid and the sphenoid sinuses. Finally, the openings of the eustachian tubes, which connect the ear and the nasopharynx, are situated directly behind the inferior turbinate.

All the sinuses pictured in Figure 5 drain into the nose, and this is very significant. If for some reason there is a marked swelling of the nasal tissues, either from infection, irritation or allergic reaction, the openings of these

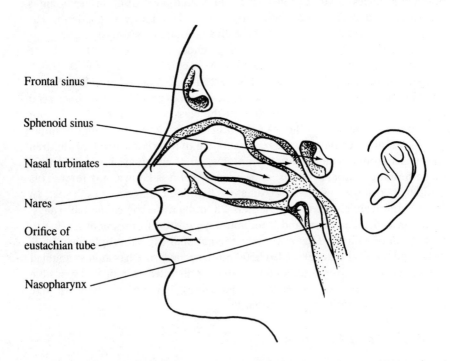

Frontal sinus

Sphenoid sinus

Nasal turbinates

Nares

Orifice of
eustachian tube

Nasopharynx

Cross section of a normal nose

sinuses can become plugged and blocked in response. Then you have trouble. One of the primary causes for such swelling is hay fever; thus sinus problems and rhinitis not infrequently go hand in hand.

Rhinitis: What Is It?

Rhinitis and sinus problems are not the same thing. The first can lead to the second, but they are decidedly two different conditions. Rhinitis means an inflammation of the mucous membranes of the nose. The condition is brought about by an allergic response, an infection or a chronic irritation of the nasal mucous membranes.

While symptoms from different causes of rhinitis may appear similar—runny nose, sneezing, and nasal irritation—it is nonetheless crucial for the doctor to differentiate between these look-alike conditions, as treatment may vary depending on the specific diagnosis. The major forms of rhinitis your child may develop include:

Seasonal allergic rhinitis   More commonly known as hay fever.

Perennial allergic rhinitis   Like hay fever but with year-round symptoms rather than seasonal ones.

Vasomotor rhinitis   This condition is caused by an imbalance in the control mechanisms that regulate the nasal mucous membranes. It is a year-round nonallergic, noninfectious form of chronic rhinitis. The nasal membranes are stimulated to overreact to such conditions as temperature changes, irritating odors and even emotional stress.

Infectious rhinitis   Another term for upper respiratory tract infections or the common cold.

Rhinitis medicamentosa   A condition caused by abuse of certain kinds of nose drops and sprays.

Seasonal allergic rhinitis Though this form of rhinitis is popularly known as hay fever or rose fever, both are misnomers; neither fever nor sensitivity to roses or hay is common to this disease. Because hay is harvested early in the farming season when ragweed pollen abounds, people once assumed it was the hay dust that caused their sneezing. Allergies to flowers of any kind, rose or otherwise, are generally quite rare, as most flower pollens are heavy and do not drift for long distances the way that mold and weed pollens do.

Allergic rhinitis is characterized by a *seasonal* pattern of recurring symptoms brought on by an allergy to the pollens of trees, grasses, weeds and mold spores. For example, in the northeastern section of the United States these reactions coincide with the appearance of tree pollen in late March and early April (see Chart 1). Grass pollens can be found in the air from early May until the beginning of July. We then have a relatively quiet time until the middle of August, when the infamous ragweed plant comes into bloom.

Chart 1. Seasonal Regional Pollen Calendar

Location	Pollen Type	Approx. Season
Alabama — Montgomery	Tree	February–April
	Grass	May–August
	Ragweed	August–October
Arizona — Phoenix	Tree	February–April
	Ragweed	September–November
	Grass	June–September
	Ragweed	March–May
	Amaranth	June–December
Arizona — Kingman	Russian Thistle—Salt Bush	July–September
	Ragweed	August–October
Arkansas — Little Rock	Tree	February–April
	Grass	May–August
	Ragweed	August–October
California — Northwestern	Tree	March–June
	Ragweed—Sage	August–December
	Grass	June–August
	Chenopod—Salt Bush	May–August
California — Southern	Tree	January–May
	Russian Thistle	August–December
	Grass	May–August
	Ragweed—Sage	August–November
California — San Francisco Bay	Tree	March–June
	Ragweed—Sage	August–November
	Grass	June–November
	Dock—Plantain	May–August
Colorado — Denver	Tree	April–June
	Sage	August–October
	Russian Thistle—Kochia	June–September
	Grass	June–August
	Ragweed	August–September
Connecticut	Tree	April–May
	Grass	May–August
	Ragweed	August–October
Delaware	Tree	April–May
	Grass	May–August
	Ragweed	August–October
District of Columbia — Washington	Tree	April–May
	Grass	May–August
	Ragweed	August–October
Florida — Miami	Tree	February–March
	Grass	April–December
	Ragweed	June–August
Florida — Tampa	Tree	March–May
	Grass	March–September
	Ragweed	August–October
Georgia — Atlanta	Tree	February–April
	Grass	May–September
	Ragweed	August–October

SOURCE: *Asthma and Allergies*, March 1980, pp. 70–73. Washington, D.C.: U.S. Department of Health and Human Services.

Chart 1. (Continued)

Location	Allergen	Jan	Feb	Mar	Apr	May	Jun	Jul	Aug	Sep	Oct	Nov	Dec
Idaho — Southern	Tree				■	■							
	Sage								■	■			
	Russian Thistle–Salt Bush							■	■	■			
	Grass					■	■	■	■				
	Ragweed								■	■			
Illinois — Chicago	Tree				■	■							
	Grass						■	■					
	Ragweed									■	■		
Indiana — Indianapolis	Tree				■	■							
	Grass						■	■					
	Ragweed									■	■		
Iowa — Ames	Tree				■	■							
	Grass						■	■	■				
	Ragweed									■	■		
Kansas — Wichita	Tree				■	■							
	Grass					■	■	■					
	Russian Thistle–Amaranth							■	■	■			
	Ragweed								■	■			
Kentucky — Louisville	Tree				■	■							
	Grass						■	■					
	Ragweed									■	■		
Louisiana — New Orleans	Tree	■	■	■									
	Grass						■	■	■	■	■	■	
	Ragweed									■	■		
Maine	Tree				■	■							
	Grass						■	■					
	Ragweed									■	■		
Maryland — Baltimore	Tree			■	■								
	Grass					■	■						
	Ragweed									■	■		
Massachusetts — Boston	Tree				■	■							
	Grass						■	■					
	Ragweed									■	■		
Michigan — Detroit	Tree				■	■							
	Grass						■	■					
	Ragweed									■	■		
Minnesota — Minneapolis	Tree				■	■							
	Chenopod–Amaranth							■	■	■			
	Grass						■	■					
	Ragweed									■	■		
Mississippi — Vicksburg	Tree			■	■								
	Grass						■	■	■				
	Ragweed									■	■		
Missouri — St. Louis, Kansas City	Tree				■	■							
	Chenopod–Amaranth							■	■	■			
	Grass						■	■					
	Ragweed									■	■		

SOURCE: *Asthma and Allergies,* March 1980, pp. 70–73. Washington, D.C.: U.S. Department of Health and Human Services.

Chart 1. (Continued)

	January	February	March	April	May	June	July	August	September	October	November	December
Montana Miles City					Tree	Grass	Russian Thistle		Ragweed—Sage			
Nebraska Omaha					Tree	Grass		Russian Thistle / Hemp	Ragweed			
Nevada Reno					Tree	Grass	Russian Thistle—Salt Bush	Sage	Ragweed			
New Hampshire					Tree	Grass			Ragweed			
New Jersey					Tree	Grass			Ragweed			
New Mexico Roswell				Tree		Grass	Amaranth—Salt Bush		Ragweed—Sage			
New York New York City					Tree	Grass			Ragweed			
North Carolina Raleigh				Tree		Grass			Ragweed			
North Dakota Fargo					Tree	Grass		Russian Thistle / Sage / Ragweed				
Ohio Cleveland					Tree	Grass			Ragweed			
Oklahoma Oklahoma City					Tree		Grass	Amaranth	Ragweed			
Oregon Portland				Tree			Grass / Dock—Plantain					
East of Cascade Mountains					Tree		Grass	Russian Thistle—Salt Bush / Sage / Ragweed				
Pennsylvania					Tree	Grass			Ragweed			

SOURCE: *Asthma and Allergies,* March 1980, pp. 70–73. Washington, D.C.: U.S. Department of Health and Human Services.

Chart 1. (Continued)

	January	February	March	April	May	June	July	August	September	October	November	December
Rhode Island				Tree								
						Grass						
									Ragweed			
South Carolina Charleston			Tree									
						Grass						
										Ragweed		
South Dakota				Tree				Russian Thistle				
						Grass			Sage			
									Ragweed			
Tennessee Nashville				Tree					Sage			
						Grass			Elm			
								Ragweed—Elm				
Texas Dallas			Tree						Sage			
						Grass						
									Ragweed			
						Grass						
Brownsville								Amaranth				
			Hackberry					Ragweed				
Utah Salt Lake City				Tree				Russian Thistle				
					Grass				Sage			
									Ragweed			
Vermont				Tree								
						Grass						
									Ragweed			
Virginia Richmond			Tree									
						Grass						
										Ragweed		
Washington Seattle			Tree									
							Grass					
						Dock—Plantain						
Eastern				Tree					Sage			
						Grass		Russian Thistle—Salt Bush				
									Ragweed			
West Virginia				Tree								
						Grass						
									Ragweed			
Wisconsin Madison				Tree								
						Grass						
									Ragweed			
Wyoming			Tree			Grass			Sage			
						Russian Thistle						
						Ragweed						

SOURCE: *Asthma and Allergies,* March 1980, pp. 70–73. Washington, D.C.: U.S. Department of Health and Human Services.

As you should know, if you have hay fever you are allergic to ragweed; the two come as a package. The pollen from this ubiquitous plant fills the air from mid-August to mid-October, reaching its peak from the last week of August to the third week of September. Even after the plant has stopped producing pollen, hay fever sufferers can sneeze until the pollen grains are killed, usually during the first hard frost. While it sometimes seems that there is no escape from ragweed's invisible army of airborne attackers, certain sections of the country are relatively ragweed free and are thus ports of refuge for many hay fever sufferers. The seashore in general and most mountain regions are usually devoid of ragweed pollen, as are deserts, especially in parts of the southwestern United States.

For many years the Southwest was a haven for seasonal rhinitis sufferers. However, during the past twenty to thirty years many people from the East and Midwest have migrated to these states. Unfortunately, they also brought with them many varieties of plants, shrubs, trees, and flowers. Now allergic rhinitis is a growing problem in these once relatively barren "pollen-free" areas.

Recognizing allergic rhinitis Clinically speaking, parents should suspect their child is suffering from seasonal allergic rhinitis if a recurring pattern of the following symptoms appears each spring, summer or early fall:

- violent sneezing spells
- itching, tearing eyes
- watery, clear, nonirritating nasal discharge
- nasal congestion, nose itching and rubbing
- reduction in the sense of smell (mostly in older children)
- mouth breathing and clearing of the throat
- complaints of itching in the ears, mouth and throat
- dark circles under the eyes during the allergic season

Keep an eye out for so-called colds that seem never to clear up. A child who suffers from these symptoms is probably the victim of allergic rhinitis rather than an infection. Table 6 provides a comparison of symptoms of the two conditions, infectious rhinitis (colds) and allergic rhinitis.

Children suffering from hay fever are especially prone to listlessness, moodiness and a kind of free-floating irritability. They may pick at their food, find fault with the world and generally become miserable to live with. When this mood descends, it is the parent's job to recognize that the change is due to a remediable physical problem and not to something intrinsically negative in the child's character. A trial period of four to seven days on an over-the-counter antihistamine or decongestant preparation is a reasonable way to deal with the problem. Examples of nonprescription drugs that may be effective include: Dimetane (an antihistamine), Chlortrimeton (an antihistamine), Sudafed (a decongestant), Afrinol (a long-acting decongestant), and Benadryl (an antihistamine).

Table 6.   Distinguishing Hay Fever from Colds

Symptom	Allergic Rhinitis	Upper Respiratory Tract Infection (URI)
Nasal discharge	Thin, watery, clear, nonirritating	Thick, yellow to green in color; local irritation
Fever	None	Low grade
Itching	In ears, nose, throat	Rarely present
Sneezing	Common in "spells"	Occasional
Nasal mucous membranes	Appear pale and swollen	Reddened, "angry" looking
Personality change	Irritable, cranky, primarily local complaints	Fatigue, generalized discomfort
Duration	Weeks to months	7 to 10 days

Carefully follow the dosage instructions printed on the package. These instructions are usually on the conservative side; up to a few years ago many over-the-counter antihistamines were prescription-only drugs. If your child's symptoms disappear while he is on the medication, no additional evaluation or treatment may be necessary. If the symptoms persist or if your child cannot tolerate these preparations, then discuss the situation with your child's physician.

Other forms of rhinitis: how to distinguish one from another   Chronic complaints of a runny or stuffy nose along with sneezing; itching of the eyes, nose or throat; a decreased sense of taste or smell and fatigue—all these symptoms may be caused by an allergy, recurring infection or vasomotor rhinitis. At times it is not an easy task for the doctor to decide why Jenny or Jack is feeling so miserable!

Perennial allergic rhinitis   The symptoms of perennial rhinitis and seasonal rhinitis (mentioned above) are the same, but perennial rhinitis is active year-round, not just during a particular pollen season. The symptoms are triggered by nonseasonal as well as seasonal allergens; dust, animal danders, wool and feathers are just a few of the many examples. One young girl I treated developed perennial rhinitis from contact with her parakeet; another from the mold spores that grew in her father's plant nursery. In general, antihistamines and decongestants may provide fairly good symptom control for most sufferers of perennial rhinitis. If you detect a direct link between the cause of the problem—the parakeet, the molds—and the symptoms, all the better. Very careful observation may be necessary to find a link, however. Keeping the child away from the cause of the symptoms is by far the best form of treatment. The child suspected of having perennial allergic rhinitis should be evaluated with the same methods used for the patient who has seasonal rhinitis.

Vasomotor or nonallergic rhinitis This condition is neither allergic nor infectious; it develops because of an apparent imbalance of the neurological control mechanisms that regulate the nasal mucous membranes. These nerves control the very rich collection of blood vessels located within the nose. If these autonomic nerves are stimulated by such challenges as changes in air temperature and humidity levels, strong, irritating odors, tobacco smoke or emotional stress, then blood flow in the nose will significantly decrease, which results in congestion of the nasal mucous membranes. Vasomotor rhinitis should be suspected when:

Nasal symptoms occur intermittently throughout the year and there is no detectable pattern of symptoms.

The most frequent complaints are nasal congestion or watery nasal discharge.

Sneezing or itching of the eyes, ears and throat are generally absent.

Sudden changes in humidity, air pressure and temperature (i.e., going from indoors to outdoors) aggravate the nasal congestion.

Strong odors, paints, perfumes, dust and cigarette smoke provoke obvious discomfort.

The treatment of vasomotor rhinitis is especially frustrating because for many people the medicines that are currently available are not particularly effective in relieving their symptoms of congestion and postnasal drip. Despite this situation it is still reasonable to try various antihistamines. They seem to be effective for some children. Over-the-counter decongestants such as pseudoephedrine or phenylpropanolamine as well as prescription drugs may also be given. Finally, if none of these preparations seem to bring relief, a nasal steroid spray such as Nasalide, Beconase or Vancenase can be prescribed by your doctor. One word of caution: follow the directions for use of these steroid sprays. Don't attempt to self-medicate your child without specific direction from your physician.

Infectious rhinitis Infectious rhinitis is primarily the result of a viral infection; in fact, it is the same as the common cold. (For a full description of the symptoms accompanying this ailment see Table 6 above.) Infectious rhinitis is present if:

The symptoms last no longer than seven to ten days.

There is, in addition to nasal congestion, a nasal discharge which varies from quite thin to very thick. This discharge is usually yellow to green in color.

The nasal secretions are quite irritating, often causing the nostrils and upper lip to become red and raw.

Other symptoms such as a cough, fever, redness of the inner nose, stomach upset and general malaise may accompany the nasal symptoms. Antihistamines and decongestants can provide some relief, but not as much as might be expected with allergic rhinitis.

Rhinitis medicamentosa There is yet another variety of rhinitis, one produced by causes somewhat different from the others. Not infrequently, in an attempt to relieve a cold or an allergic nasal condition, over-the-counter decongestant nose drops or sprays may be used for many weeks at a time. Prolonged application of these drugs is an abuse, and when this occurs the medication which is supposed to control symptoms ends up making them a good deal worse. As the effectiveness of the decongestant declines and the symptoms become increasingly severe, the patient, in the true mode of the addict, comes to depend on larger and larger doses of the medicine to get relief from symptoms now being caused by the drug rather than the original condition. This situation is known as rhinitis medicamentosa. Freely translated the name means "The medicine did it."

Here is a typical scenario: Amy has a runny nose and is constantly sniffling. Her mother goes to the pharmacy and selects one of the many brands of nonprescription nose drops or sprays on display. This medicine is given according to the instructions on the label and at first it seems to decrease if not entirely eliminate Amy's congestion. After four or five days it seems that the drops must be given more frequently because the symptomatic relief Amy experiences has become increasingly shorter. Before too long, Amy's mother is giving her child doses of the spray two times a day, then four, then eight, then in desperation ten, then more. And still the condition refuses to improve.

What to do? Simple. Throw the nose drops or sprays into the garbage *immediately!* Unless medication is halted on the spot the symptoms will continue to worsen, and the possibility of permanent damage to the child's nasal mucous membranes will increase proportionately. Some time ago a nineteen-year-old pregnant woman who had been suffering from chronic nasal congestion for almost two years came to my office. Despite medication her condition was getting worse all the time. When I asked what drugs she was using, she dug into her pocketbook and produced an over-the-counter nasal spray, announcing that she had been going through a bottle of this medicine *every two days,* and that she had been following this regime for *eighteen straight months.* The woman, it turned out, was addicted to her decongestant. The only way to get her "unhooked" was to substitute a cortisone nasal spray for the present medication, and at that, the weaning process was a slow and difficult one. Moral: never use over-the-counter nasal preparations carelessly and *never* use them for more than four or five days at a time. If your child shows any signs of becoming dependent on such preparations, even when they are employed only occasionally, discontinue their use right away and consult your physician.

Treatment for Rhinitis

Once a diagnosis has been reached based on history, physical findings and appropriate laboratory tests, recommendations for your child's rhinitis condition will be made. As with the other conditions we have discussed, treatment falls into three broad headings: pharmacotherapy, environmental control measures and immunotherapy.

Pharmacotherapy

While most people associate the symptomatic treatment of allergic rhinitis with antihistamines and decongestants alone, a relatively new prophylactic agent, cromolyn sodium, known commercially as Nasalcrom, plus, several cortisone nasal preparations are important players on the therapeutic team. Let's have a look at these medications in more detail.

ANTIHISTAMINES   When we refer to an antihistamine, we are actually speaking of six different chemical groups within the same pharmaceutical family, all of them possessing antihistaminic properties. What exactly are these properties?

Antihistamines neutralize the effects of histamine, the chemical mediator responsible for causing many of the typical symptoms associated with allergy. Antihistamines accomplish this by blocking areas called receptor sites located on the surface of cells. If histamine, which is responsible for the sneezing, itchy eyes and runny nose of chronic rhinitis, is prevented from reaching these receptor sites, effective symptom control can be accomplished.

An important point to remember in this process is that antihistamines work best *before* the histamine is released into the blood, that is, before the allergic reaction has gotten started, and this is clearly the most efficient way to take this medicine—before the symptoms begin. (For more detailed information regarding the workings of histamine see page x.) Antihistamines are a rather diverse collection of drugs divided into six different groups or families. Since a drug from one of these families may be effective in providing relief for one child but not for another, it's possible that your doctor will try several different varieties of antihistamine before the best one is found. Once the most effective medication is determined, it can then be used for extended periods.

A few notes on the antihistamines Liquid antihistamines are absorbed into the bloodstream rapidly and tend to go to work faster than either capsules or tablets. Whenever there is an urgent need for an antihistamine, the liquid form is your best bet.

Small children have difficulty swallowing tablets and capsules. For those under two years of age, liquid antihistamines are the preferred form.

If your child requires daily doses of an antihistamine for an extended period of time, a long-acting tablet or capsule medication is the best form in which to administer the drug. Common sense tells us that taking medicine twice a day is a more efficient method of drug delivery than dosing it every six hours or four times a day.

When beginning a course of antihistamines, be alert to the development of side effects. While drowsiness is the most common of these, it is often mild and tends not to interfere with the child's normal functioning. If extreme drowsiness or any other side effects mentioned above become a problem, discontinue the medicine and contact your doctor immediately. Your doctor will most likely switch your child to another antihistamine.

Over a period of weeks to months some children may develop a tolerance for a certain antihistamine. When this occurs, the medication will no longer be effective and another must be substituted. Armed with this knowledge, you should not be surprised if your doctor changes antihistamine prescriptions, as this switching is a normal part of rhinitis therapy. Interestingly enough, after some time has passed, the child may then return to the original antihistamine and discover that it again works as well as it did before the medicine was switched.

Despite what some people may tell you, there is no one "best" antihistamine. The best antihistamine is the one that works best for your child. Period.

Table 7 gives an overview of how antihistamine drugs are organized. The possible side effects of all these drugs include sleepiness, gastrointestinal upset, a jittery feeling, and sometimes hyperactivity.

DECONGESTANTS Decongestants are vasoconstricting agents, and as such they cause a narrowing of the blood vessels in the nasal mucous membranes that decreases the swelling and congestion found in most forms of rhinitis. These medicines can cause unpleasant side effects; children using them must be carefully watched. Specific decongestant agents include pseudoephedrine hydrochloride, ephedrine, phenylpropanolamine, pseudoephedrine SO_4 and phenylepherine. Decongestants are available in a variety of forms including liquids, tablets, nasal sprays and drops. They are often combined with an antihistamine into a single preparation, as shown in Table 8.

Among decongestants, the nose drops and spray forms are the most frequently used and abused. Therefore both for children and parents, *never use a decongestant spray or nose drop for longer than five days in a row.*

Why? Recall the pregnant woman who was addicted to decongestants. After four or five days, most topical decongestants' effective duration of action decreases considerably, so that the medicine must be administered at shorter and shorter intervals to bring relief. Eventually, through what is called a rebound mechanism, the drops or sprays begin to *cause* the nasal congestion the decongestant was designed to inhibit; at the same time the user becomes increasingly dependent on the drug, using greater and greater amounts to achieve ever less and less relief. This condition, as mentioned, is called rhinitis medicamentosa. Treatment consists of discontinuing topical nasal prepara-

Table 7. Antihistamine Overview

Generic Name	Brand Name	Available Forms
Ethanolamines		
Carbinoxamine maleate	Clistin	Tablets, elixir
	Rondec	Tablets, drops, syrup, sustained-release tablet
Clemastine fumarate	Tavist	Tablets
	Tavist-1	Tablets
Diphenhydramine HCl*	Benadryl	Capsules, elixir
Doxylamine succinate	Decapryn	Tablets, syrup
	Formula 44*	Cough mixture
	Vicks Nyquil*	Cough mixture
Phenyltoloxamine citrate	Naldecon	Tablets, syrup, drops
	Sinutab*	Tablets
	Sinubid*	Tablets
Ethylenediamines		
Pyrilamine maleate	Triaminic preparations	
Pyrilamine tannate	Rynatan	Tablets, pediatric suspension
Tripelennamine HCl	Pyribenzamine (PBZ)	Sustained-release tablet
Tripelennamine citrate	PBZ	Elixir
Alkylamines		
Brompheniramine maleate	Dimetane*	Tablets, elixir, sustained-release tablet
	Dimetapp	Elixir, sustained-release tablet
Chlorpheniramine maleate	A.R.M.*	Tablets
	Allerest*	Chewable tablets
	Chlor-Trimeton*	Tablets, syrup, sustained-release repetabs
	Contac*	Capsules
	Coricidin*	Tablets
	Deconamine	Tablets, elixir, sustained-release capsules
	Demazin	Syrup, sustained-release tablet
	Dristan*	Tablets

Table 7. *(Continued)*

Generic Name	Brand Name	Available Forms
	Fedahist	Tablets, syrup, sustained-release tablet
	Isoclor	Tablets, syrup, sustained-release tablet
	Naldecon preparations	
	Novafed A	Capsules, syrup
	Sudafed-Plus	Tablets, syrup
	Teldrin	Sustained-release capsule
Chlorpheniramine tannate	Rynatan	Tablets, pediatric suspension
Dexbrompheniramine maleate	Disophrol	Sustained-release tablet
	Drixoral	Sustained-release tablet
Dexchlorpheniramine maleate	Polaramine	Sustained-release tablets, syrup
Triprolidine HCl	Actidil	Tablets, syrup
	Actifed	Tablets, syrup
Piperazines		
Hydroxyzine HCl	Atarax	Tablets, pediatric suspension
Hydroxyzine pamoate	Vistaril	Capsules, syrup
Meclizine HCl	Antivert	Tablets
	Bonine	Chewable tablets
Phenothiazines		
Methdilazine HCl	Tacaryl	Tablets, syrup
Promethazine HCl	Phenergan	Tablets, syrup
Trimeprazine tartrate	Temaril	Tablets, syrup, sustained-release capsule
Piperidines		
Azatadine maleate	Optimine	Tablets
Cyproheptadine HCl	Periactin	Tablets, syrup
Peripheral H_1 Antagonist Terfenadine†	Seldane	Tablets

NOTE: Discuss with your doctor the dose appropriate for your child.
*Over-the-counter preparation.
†This preparation is the first antihistamine with little or no sleep-producing effects.

tions immediately. In other words, if five or more days of use have already elapsed, throw away those drops and sprays *right now.*

Side effects In general, decongestant sprays and drops cause fewer general or systemic side effects than orally administered decongestants. When side effects do occur, typical symptoms include:

nausea
dizziness
nervousness
tachycardia (rapid heartbeat)
hyperactive behavior
transient (temporary) high or low blood pressure, and/or irregular heart-
    beat (such reactions are unusual and are generally limited to young
    children; stopping the medicine immediately will cause these reac-
    tions to cease)

CROMOLYN SODIUM: NASALCROM AND OPTICROM   Cromolyn sodium has the unique ability to block allergic reactions *before* they occur. If it worked for every patient, I could spend all my time writing books because no one would visit my office with allergic symptoms. Unfortunately, for allergy suffer-ers there is no single drug currently available that comes even close to being 100 percent effective, cromolyn included. Still, this useful medication is the first example of a prophylactic drug for rhinitis or conjunctivitis, and the good news is that researchers tell us that others will soon follow.

Two forms of cromolyn sodium are available for the prevention of allergic eye and nasal symptoms: Opticrom and Nasalcrom. Both must be used four times a day at the beginning of treatment, either one drop of Opticrom in each eye or one spray of Nasalcrom in each nostril. Clinical benefits from this drug may be detected as early as three to four days after treatment has started, or as late as the third or fourth week. When a positive response takes place, the dosage can then be decreased to three and perhaps even two times a day. Cromolyn does not relieve symptoms once they are present; it must be used on a daily basis before problems arise.

Side effects Cromolyn has been proven to be an extremely safe prepara-tion that can be administered on a regular basis for long periods of time. The potential side effects, though ordinarily minimal, may include:

sneezing
transient burning of the nasal mucous membranes
headaches
a bad taste in the mouth

These symptoms, when they do occur, are generally not serious and tend to disappear when the medication is discontinued. Really, the major problem

Table 8.   Antihistamine/Decongestant Overview

Name	Available	Antihistamine	Decongestant
Actifed	Prescription	Triprolidine HCl	Pseudoephedrine HCl
Clistin-D	Prescription	Carbinoxamine maleate	Phenylepherine HCl
Contac	Over the counter	Chlorpheniramine maleate	Phenylpropanol-amine HCl
Deconamine	Prescription	Chlorpheniramine maleate	Pseudoephedrine HCl
Dimetapp	Prescription	Brompheniramine maleate	Phenylepherine HCl Phenylpropanol-amine HCl
Dristan	Over the counter	Chlorpheniramine maleate	Phenylepherine HCl
Isoclor	Prescription	Chlorpheniramine maleate	Pseudoephedrine HCl
Naldecon	Prescription	Chlorpheniramine maleate Phenyltoloxamine citrate	Phenylpropanol-amine HCl Phenylepherine HCl
Novahistine	Over the counter	Chlorpheniramine maleate	Phenylpropanol-amine HCl
Ornade	Over the counter	Chlorpheniramine maleate	Phenylpropanol-amine HCl
Rondec	Prescription	Carbinoxamine maleate	Pseudoephedrine HCl
Rynatan	Prescription	Chlorpheniramine tannate Pyrilamine tannate	Phenylepherine tannate
Sinubid	Prescription	Phenyltoloxamine citrate	Phenylpropanol-amine HCl
Sudafed-Plus	Over the counter	Chlorpheniramine maleate	Pseudoephedrine HCl
Triaminic	Over the counter	Pyrilamine maleate Pheniramine maleate	Phenylpropanol-amine HCl

Table 9.   Commonly Used Nasal Decongestants

Generic Name	Brand Name	Available Form
Pseudoephedrine HCl	Novafed	Liquid, capsules
	Sudafed	Tablets, syrup
Pseudoephedrine SO$_4$	Afrinol	Sustained-release tablet
Phenylepherine HCl	Coricidin	Spray
	Neo-Synephrine	Spray, drops
Phenylpropanolamine HCl	Propadrine HCl	Capsules, elixir
Naphazoline HCl	Privine HCl	Spray, drops
Oxymetazoline HCl	Afrin	Spray, drops
Tetrahydrozoline HCl	Tyzine	Spray, drops
Xylometazoline HCl	Neo-Synephrine II	Spray, drops
	Otrivin	Spray, drops
	Sinutab Sinus	Spray

NOTE: Neither drops nor sprays should be used for more than five days; then the decongestant *must* be discontinued.

with cromolyn is less one of side effects and more one of compliance and human error; even the most efficient parents sometimes forget to make sure their children take the drug on a regular four-times-a-day schedule, and the children themselves either cannot be bothered or are incapable of medicating themselves. Yet without faithful adherence to the recommended treatment directions, cromolyn will simply not work effectively.

What's more, while cromolyn treatment is advisable for any child suffering from vasomotor or allergic rhinitis, it by no means works for everyone, and only after a period of at least four weeks can a decision be made regarding its effectiveness for your child. If your child is about to start using cromolyn sodium, look upon the chances of success with bright optimism but not with blind hope.

STEROIDS   These drugs, which are derived from powerful, naturally occurring hormones produced by the adrenal glands, are potent anti-inflammatory agents. They are highly effective for the treatment of chronic rhinitis because of their ability to decrease local swelling. Their major drawback is the fact that when used for a prolonged period they can produce serious and in some situations even life-threatening side effects. They are in effect the proverbial double-edged sword.

Any steroid taken by mouth in large doses for weeks at a time will cause unwanted complications. Fortunately, within the past five years, two topically active, poorly absorbed cortisone derivatives, beclomethasone dipropionate and flunisolide, have become commercially available. These drugs are marketed as: Beconase or Vancenase (beclomethasone dipropionate), which comes in a gas-propelled dispenser, and Nasalide (flunisolide), which is in pump-spray container.

Either of these preparations can be used for weeks at a time in the appropriately prescribed dose without fear of dangerous side effects. Two complaints that occur with some frequency are a transient burning sensation immediately after using the spray and less often the development of a bloody nose. If either of these situations develop, contact your doctor right away for new instructions.

Beconase and Vancenase have been approved by the FDA for children aged twelve or older. Nasalide is recommended for youngsters down to the age of six.

For any child who continues to have significant rhinitis symptoms despite treatment with antihistamines, decongestants and cromolyn, a trial with either of these cortisone derivatives is in order. Discuss the appropriate starting dose with your child's doctor.

A treatment for chronic rhinitis among ear, nose and throat specialists is a procedure involving injection of a long-acting steroid preparation directly into the nasal turbinates. *This technique can on rare occasions cause extremely dangerous side effects.* Given the fact that efficient topically active steroid preparations and/or quick bursts of oral steroids are available for children suffering from severe rhinitis, it is my opinion that the use of nasal steroid injections should be discouraged, if not abandoned entirely. If a doctor suggests such a procedure for your child, I advise that you get a second opinion before consenting to this treatment.

Environmental Control Measures

The easiest, cheapest, most painless way to relieve allergic symptoms is to simply remove the substance and/or allergen responsible for causing the problem, provided, of course, you have the luxury of knowing what the substance is. If you do, then you can practice the simplest antiallergy measure of all: environmental control. Henry's runny nose, tearing eyes and itchy throat are, we know, due to a family cat. You can solve the problem quickly by removing the cat from the premises. A horsehair sofa in the den makes Judy sneeze and sniffle. Replace it with a couch filled with a nonallergenic stuffing. Feathers are Larry's nemesis. Give that pet bird away to a friend or relative and get rid of all down comforters and pillows. In many cases it really is just as easy as that. Here are some practical steps you can take in this direction.

Humidification In areas of the country where heating is needed and especially in homes where forced-air heating is used, the air generally becomes exceedingly dry and irritating to the nose, mouth and throat. This dryness bothers just about everyone but is especially troublesome for children with chronic nasal congestion. In a house that has low relative humidity (less than 35 percent) a sleeping child who is a mouth breather will awaken with complaints of a sore throat. Typically, this problem is worse on arising and improves dramatically as the day progresses, only to recur the next morning! The problem stems not from a virus or a bacteria, but from a simple lack of adequate humidity in the air.

The remedy is simple: increase the amount of water vapor in the air. The optimal relative humidity for your home is between 35 and 45 percent, and you can raise it to this level by a variety of means. One no-frills method is to simply fill pans with water and place them near the heating units in every room of the house. The passive evaporation of the water will soon increase the level of the relative humidity in the air and your child should quickly feel the difference.

More sophisticated are the various electronic humidifiers and vaporizers on the market today. The most efficient of these is the *ultrasonic cool mist humidifier.* This space age appliance uses sound waves to produce a superfine vapor of mist that remains suspended in the air for a long time. This humidifier manufactures water droplets so small they easily penetrate deep into a child's mouth, throat and lungs. A fringe benefit of the ultrasonic humidifier is that the water vapor is so finely dispersed throughout the atmosphere that floors, walls and bedding do not end up being drenched; the older models are not always so obliging. Sound too good to be true? Well, there is one significant drawback: cost. The usual retail price for this machine is from $50 to $150. Not cheap. Still, careful shoppers will look for ultrasonic humidifiers on sale at the end of the summer season. As these units become increasingly popular, market competition will no doubt work its magic and drive the prices down to a more generally affordable level.

A word on steam vaporizers: while useful for children who suffer from croup and sinusitis, these devices are, in my experience, practically worthless as far as rhinitis is concerned. Hot air vaporizers may stimulate the growth of allergy-causing molds in and around the child's living area, and in some instances the warm steam from these appliances irritates the rhinitis condition rather than soothes it. Relatedly, there is no medical reason that I know of for adding inhalants such as eucalyptus, Vicks Vaporub and menthol to a vaporizer. Though these substances bring a pleasing medicinal odor to the immediate atmosphere and perhaps create the illusion that they are "cleaning out" the lungs, in truth they serve no therapeutic purpose.

Dust control Dust is the accumulation of the breakdown products of all the organic materials found in the home. The dust in my home will be different from the dust in your home, depending on how each is furnished and the life-style of its occupants. A family that owns several pets, likes to keep their windows open, and has wool carpeting throughout the house will have a substantially different type of dust from the folks next door who use central air conditioning, keep no pets and have synthetic fiber carpets.

Chief, perhaps, of the allergens in dust is the so-called *dust mite,* a microscopically tiny creature that lives in every house, specifically in every bed. Unlike bedbugs, dust mites are not limited to homes of poor hygiene or poverty. Comfortably ensconced in pillows and mattresses, this ubiquitous animal derives its nourishment from the dead skin cells that flake off our bodies during the hours of rest. Vacuuming the mattress and mattress cover when the bed linens are changed and putting your pillows in a clothes dryer every few weeks will significantly reduce the dust mite population.

There are a number of other measures you can take to monitor dust control.

All carpets should be frequently vacuumed. When buying carpets, choose those of synthetic fibers with low-pile construction. Vacuum all carpets every two to three days.

All dustable surfaces should be gone over two to three times a week, especially in the bedrooms. Make sure that your allergic child is not in the area when you clean.

Bedroom closets should be used only for clothes that are worn on a regular basis. Seasonally stored clothes should be kept in a separate area, preferably in a cellar, attic or in dry storage. If seasonal items must be stored in the bedroom closet, keep them in garment bags and dust them periodically.

Window shades or washable curtains in the bedroom are preferable to louvered blinds and heavy drapes.

The dilemma of what to do concerning a family pet that is known to cause an allergy provides the family with a difficult situation. Obviously the answer is to remove the animal as quickly as possible. That's the easy part. But to suddenly give away a beloved animal, "a relative of my whole family" as one young man described his bulldog to me, is asking a lot of a child. I have come to prefer a step-by-step solution to this nettlesome problem. First banish the dog or cat from the child's section of the house. Then see if the allergy symptoms improve. Sometimes this change alone will be all that's necessary. If step one doesn't bring substantial symptom relief, try restricting the animal to a single room in the house. Then observe the effect. If the previous steps fail, remove the animal from the house entirely, making a home for it in the garage or in an outbuilding. If all else fails, then and then only should you think of finding the animal another home.

Even this last step can have the sting somewhat softened by applying a similar step-by-step approach. 1. Prepare the child ahead of time, gently explaining why and how the animal will have to be given away. Do not simply snatch the creature up one day and whisk it off without a warning. 2. Find the pet a good home. 3. Make sure the child knows where this home will be, that it will be benevolent, that the pet's new masters will be caring. 4. Be certain the child understands that all this is being done not as a punishment but as a sad and necessary step toward helping the situation. 5. Substitute a nonallergenic pet for the old one. Gerbils, hamsters, guinea pigs, turtles, fish or even snakes are possible replacements.

If your home is heated with a forced-air type heating system, place filters over the out-flow registers. Several layers of cheesecloth make a fine homemade filter, though commercial air conditioning filters are a bit more efficient and neat.

A centrally installed humidifier will help control dry air syndrome. A humidistat can also be used to record relative humidity throughout the house and to determine the efficiency of your humidification unit.

A variety of mechanical devices can be used to filter the air of pollen, dander, dust and smoke fumes, the two basic types being electrostatic precipitators and electronic filters. Of the electronic filters the HEPA filter is best, primarily because it does not generate potentially irritating ozone gas as do a number of electrostatic filter devices. The most efficient (and most expensive) HEPA units are centrally installed into forced-air heating systems. An alternative is to use single, freestanding HEPA filter units in the principal rooms of your house, especially in the allergic child's bedroom. Any air conditioning professional will be able to fill you in on the details.

Immunotherapy

Immunotherapy, or as it is sometimes called, "desensitization," "hyposensitization" or "allergy shots," is a method in which a patient is given a regular course of injections containing the allergens to which she is clinically allergic. The usual course of treatment lasts from two to four years and the injections are generally continued until the patient has become symptom free without the need for medication for a 12- to 15-month period. Response to treatment usually takes at least three to six months to become apparent, and parents should not expect to see signs of improvement before this time.

For treatment of seasonal allergic rhinitis, immunotherapy has proven to be quite effective. If a child has an allergic problem which is present only during a single season of the year and if he is sensitive to only one or two particular plants or trees, this child should respond quite well to immunotherapy. On the other hand, a child who has multiple sensitivities, who has been allergic for many years, and who remains symptomatic all year round has less chance of a successful outcome. This does not mean that the latter patient cannot be helped, only that his possibilities of a good response are somewhat less than those of the former.

While there is definite evidence that injection treatment is effective for children allergic to specific pollens, response rates for patients sensitive to allergens such as dust, molds and animal dander are still being evaluated. It is my opinion that at present immunotherapy for food allergy is ineffectual and should be avoided. For a more detailed description on the mechanics of immunotherapy, see page 42.

Complications That May Occur from Rhinitis

Although the symptoms of chronic rhinitis are considered to be primarily annoying rather than serious, complications can develop which can be quite serious.

Sinusitis From a developmental point of view there is no general agreement among medical scientists regarding the role of the sinuses. What are they exactly? No one is sure. There are four pairs of sinuses—the maxillary, ethmoid, frontal and sphenoid (see Figure 5). It has been suggested that these areas are somehow involved with our sense of smell and the production of protective mucus secretions. They also probably play a role in some aspects of voice control and, because they are hollow, their structure reduces the total weight of the head.

The inner surfaces of the sinuses are lined with millions of tiny hairs that regularly propel mucus secretions out of the hollow spaces inside the sinuses, thereby cleaning, lubricating and maintaining these delicate areas in sound working order. Located behind the nose and eyes, sinuses are connected to the nasal passageways by means of tiny openings that allow air to enter and mucus to drain out.

Normally you are not aware of your sinuses until an allergic reaction develops involving the membranes of the nose. At this moment the sinus membranes, which are really a continuation of the nasal membranes, can swell violently and overflow with mucus, blocking the drainage openings leading into the nose. Fluids then become trapped in the passageways, causing a buildup of pressure which eventually can lead to painful, sometimes overpowering headaches. The trapped mucus, meanwhile, becomes an ideal place for viruses and bacteria to set up housekeeping, the end result being a sinus infection (sinusitis), which may include chills, fever, dizziness, severe headaches and thick greenish mucus.

Treatment for sinusitis consists of oral decongestants, antihistamines, and, when infection is present, antibiotics. Topical nasal preparations in the form of drops or sprays used to shrink the membranes and dry the mucus secretions should not be used for more than five days.

If your child seems to be having discomfort caused by sinus involvement and you are unable to get to the doctor, here are some temporary home remedies:

Have the child inhale steam from a vaporizer or a pot of boiling water. *Never* leave your child unattended around boiling water or a steam vaporizer. In the blink of an eye a scalding can take place.

The application of a moist heated compress over the sinus areas may temporarily help relieve some pain and pressure. All these remedies are temporary, of course, and should by no means be used to replace adequate medical attention.

In the unusual event of recurring sinus infections that cannot be brought under control with appropriate antibiotic therapy, some form of surgery may be required. In children the most common procedure is called a nasal antrostomy. This operation provides a permanent drainage pathway from the infected sinus into the nose, making it impossible for the mucus to accumulate and become reinfected. This procedure is rarely necessary.

Nosebleeds Any time a child has a problem with chronic nasal symptoms, the possibility of nosebleeds (epistaxis) increases. Children suffering from the irritation of chronic rhinitis will often pick at and bore into their nostrils with a vengeance, despite all pleas and protestations from their parents. Eventually the constant trauma to the delicate nasal membranes causes superficial blood vessels to rupture, especially those located on the nasal septum dividing the wall between the nostrils. A bloody nose is the inevitable result.

Nosebleeds tend to occur with increased frequency during the colder months of the year when household heating dries out the linings of the nose. All it may take at this point is a minor shock—a strong sneeze, for example —to break the superficial vessels and start the blood flowing. Such nosebleeds are not serious, of course, but they can be irksome to the parents and frightening to the child. If frequent bleeding continues even after you have increased the humidity level in your home, a visit to an ear, nose and throat specialist may eventually be necessary. More than likely the doctor will solve the problem by applying a chemical or an electric probe to the superficial vessel that has been bleeding. This is a simple, painless procedure that is usually quite effective.

Changes in the dental arch Children who suffer from constant nasal congestion often become chronic mouth breathers. If unchecked, this condition can cause a permanent change in the shape of the mouth that results in the formation of a high-arched palate and changes in the dental arch. Children who are possible candidates for these problems are easily recognized. Perhaps you have seen these children in nursery school or playing in the park. They constantly breathe through their mouths and have persistent nasal congestion or a continually runny nose. The major problem that develops because of the rhinitis is malocclusion of the upper and lower jaws. Unless the chronic nasal problem is treated aggressively, extensive orthodontic work may be required to correct the dental condition.

Questions and Answers about Rhinitis

How severe can hay fever become?

While hay fever is hardly fatal, some children are made so uncomfortable that they become prisoners in their own homes during pollen season. They are less efficient at school, more irritable, and in general quite miserable. Hay-fever symptoms run the gamut from being a mere annoyance to becoming an intransigent, if temporary, agony. Happily, with appropriate medical care almost all children can be helped.

If left untreated, will rhinitis symptoms tend to disappear or will they continue indefinitely?

There are certainly untreated children who, over a period of time, lose their allergic sensitivity and their nasal symptoms. There is no way of knowing whether your child will be among these lucky ones. Very often pediatricians tell parents that their child will outgrow her allergic problem within the next "several" years and that specific treatment is therefore unnecessary. The reality is that certain children afflicted with allergic rhinitis get better on their own, some get worse, some stay the same. The decision to seek medical advice for a child who has chronic or recurrent rhinitis symptoms should depend on the duration and severity of the complaints.

What will happen if a child's rhinitis condition is allowed to go medically untreated?

At best you will have a very unhappy young person on your hands plus a family that has become utterly frustrated by the child's endless sneezing and complaining. Also, if the symptoms of chronic rhinitis are too long ignored, they might be the forerunner of lower respiratory tract symptoms such as wheezing and difficulty in breathing. This condition does not develop very frequently, contrary to what some doctors may tell parents to scare them into action, but why take the chance?

When parents purchase over-the-counter decongestants or antihistamines, should they ask for these medicines in children's strengths?

Yes. Most antihistamines and decongestants are available in pediatric strengths. The pharmacist or your doctor will give you guidance in this area.

Which forms of medication are preferable for children, nose drops or sprays?

Most children tolerate nasal sprays better than drops. Decongestant drops are difficult to administer, for one thing. They almost always "leak" from the nose into the throat where their bitter taste makes children quite understandably grimace and complain. A nasal spray is easier to use. The child does not have to lie down—standing is, in fact, the preferred position for taking a spray. Sprays in general deliver a more diffuse application of the medicine over the surface of the nasal membranes. I cannot remind you too often not to allow your child to use a topical nasal decongestant, either in spray form or drops, for more than five days in a row.

Does aspirin help rhinitis?

No, not on its own. If a headache happens to accompany a rhinitis attack, as it occasionally does, the aspirin will probably help relieve it. It will *not* reduce the primary symptoms of the rhinitis itself.

Why do some allergic children develop dark circles under their eyes?

These dark circles are popularly known as "allergic shiners." They are not due to lack of sleep or poor eating habits but are produced by the slow movement of blood, which collects in the capillary beds under the eyes. The blood flow is slowed by the allergic swelling that occurs in the nasal mucous membranes. The darkness itself is due to a "pooling" of venous blood that accumulates in these thin-walled superficial blood vessels under the eyes. During the times of year when a child has allergic symptoms, he may develop these shiners on a fairly regular basis. They have no sinister significance. When the season passes and swelling in the nose recedes, they will disappear. Allergic shiners are nothing to be alarmed about and in no way indicate any underlying pathology, except for the allergic condition.

At what age can the symptoms of allergic rhinitis begin?

In theory, rhinitis can start at any age. The youngest rhinitis patient I can recall was a five-day-old infant named David who was allergic to his formula and developed severe nasal obstruction. When a nonmilk formula was introduced into David's diet, his nasal symptoms disappeared. In practice this case is quite unusual because of the exceptionally early onset of symptoms. Typically, seasonal allergic symptoms appear only after a child has become sensitized to aeroallergens such as trees, grass or weed pollens, a process of exposure that ordinarily takes several years before symptoms become apparent.

What part, if any, do stress and emotional anxiety play in the development of rhinitis?

In my opinion the development of *allergic* rhinitis is not influenced by emotional factors. Some forms of chronic rhinitis, specifically vasomotor rhinitis, can and quite often will be aggravated by periods of stress and anxiety.

Are there particular times of day when a child's rhinitis becomes better or worse?

Seasonal rhinitis sufferers generally have their most intense symptoms in the early morning and in the late afternoon or early evening. These are the times of the day when plants usually release their pollen into the air.

Can houseplants cause allergic rhinitis?

Rarely. The only potential problem may be found in the soil. Occasionally, molds that thrive in potting soil can irritate the allergies of highly mold sensitive children. On the whole, for the majority of children nonflowering houseplants are nothing to worry about.

Teachers will sometimes insist that a child suffering from chronic rhinitis actually has a cold and should be kept out of school. How should parents deal with such a situation?

If a child is diagnosed as having an allergic problem, either of a seasonal or year-round nature, the doctor should provide you with a note to this effect; the note should then be sent on to the proper school authorities. The real difficulty comes at those times when the child develops a cold *superimposed* on an underlying allergic condition and it becomes difficult to tell the two apart. In such situations there are still certain criteria that can be applied:

If the child has a fever, she should be kept home.

If mucus coming from the child's nose is thick and yellowish, an infection is most likely the cause of the symptoms, not an allergy.

If the child complains of symptoms such as aches and pains, a viral infection may be present.

Hives and Angioedema

Hives (urticaria) Anyone who has ever been plagued by hives or who has stood helplessly by and watched a family member suffer the relentless itching (pruritis) this ailment brings will agree that hives can literally drive a person mad. Some of the most uncomfortable and troubled patients I have seen over the past twenty years have been victims of this most unpleasant condition.

Appearing on the surface of the skin as well-outlined raised areas, hives tend to have a whitish or reddish coloration. There is no typical size for the lesions themselves; they can be as small as a pencil eraser or large enough to cover an entire arm or leg. Similarly, there is no specific part of the body more prone to hives than any other; we are susceptible from the tops of our heads to the bottoms of our feet, and it is even possible to develop lesions internally along the length of the intestinal tract. An attack of hives can consist of one large hive, several hives located in different parts of the body, or a cluster of many small hives concentrated in a specific area. Sometimes individual welts will "grow together," forming a single large, irregularly shaped swelling which covers a large section of the body. Lesions of this size are known as giant hives.

The itching sensation associated with hives is the most disheartening part of it all. I have seen infants practically tear their skin off in a futile attempt to find relief. The localized itching and swelling of hives is caused by the leakage of fluids from the smallest blood vessels located just beneath the surface of the skin after histamine is released during an allergic reaction.

As a rule, an eruption of hives appears without warning, makes the child intensely uncomfortable for several hours, then slowly subsides. Occasionally, though, hives may be present for considerably longer, sometimes for months or even years. Technically speaking, hives that recur for six weeks or more are defined as chronic; six weeks or less, acute. The chance of determining the actual cause of acute hives is less than 30 percent, while for a chronic condition the percentage decreases to under 10 percent. Fortunately in both situations, while the origin is difficult to determine, medical relief of symptoms is usually within reach.

It is estimated that 10 to 20 percent of the American population will at one time or another suffer from an episode of hives. Acute urticaria tends to appear more frequently among people who are allergic; chronic hives strikes the allergic and nonallergic child with equal frequency.

Angioedema   Simply stated, angioedema represents a hive that has invaded the deeper skin layers. The swelling of angioedema is usually more spread out and less distinct. A big difference between hives and angioedema is that the first one itches and the second one doesn't. The persistent itching so closely associated with hives occurs because the nerves transmitting the "itch sensation" are located in the outermost skin layers where the hives develop. Angioedema, on the other hand, rarely produces itching, as the superficial free nerve endings are not affected. Indeed, it is the extreme swelling associated with angioedema that may occasionally cause pain rather than itching, especially if the swelling occurs in areas of the body where the skin is tightly stretched, such as on the fingers.

While hives can certainly drive you to distraction, they rarely, if ever, are the cause of a potentially life-threatening situation. Angioedema, on the other hand, if it involves areas such as the tongue, mouth or windpipe (trachea), may prove to be fatal if it continues without appropriate medical attention.

The Physiology of Hives

Hives develop when the chemical mediator histamine is secreted into the bloodstream and body tissues. This substance can be released by several different mechanisms, the most common being an allergic reaction. Regardless of the triggering factor, the end result of histamine in the superficial skin layers is the same: leakage of fluid out of the small blood vessels, localized swelling, the consequent production of wheals, and the all-too-familiar sensation of unrelenting itching. (For a detailed description of the mechanism of histamine release and the part it plays in the allergic process, see page 9.)

Mysteries remain, of course, as to how this entire process works. To date, researchers have been unable to prove that histamine is the only mediator involved in hive formation; there may well be others we have not yet discovered. The question of why certain children develop allergic responses while others do not remains one of the enduring riddles in allergy research.

Helping Your Doctor Diagnose the Cause of Hives

Hives and angioedema are usually easy to identify; discovering the causes behind them is far more difficult. You can help by becoming a careful observer and by keeping a watchful eye out for answers to the following pertinent questions, many of which you will be asked at the time of your child's first medical consultation.

When do the hives appear?

On what parts of the body are they located?

How long do they last? Do they tend to come and go or do they remain for prolonged periods of time?

Describe their size and appearance.

How frequently do they occur? What are the average time intervals that separate each attack?

Under what particular circumstances, if any, do they seem to occur?

Are any unusual circumstances present when the rash appears?

What foods has the child eaten in the twenty-four-hour period preceding the onset? (Be alert for new or unusual foods that have recently been introduced, especially those that classically cause allergic responses—chocolate, eggs, citrus fruits, shellfish, strawberries, wheat, nuts and milk.)

Has there been recent exposure at school or at home to unusual substances: chemicals, pesticides, hobby paints and glues, industrial materials?

Has the child recently experienced added emotional stress owing to conflicts with friends, family, school situations, general life circumstances? Do the hives tend to appear after periods of excitement or temper tantrums?

What is the current state of the child's overall health? Is he convalescing from any long-term ailment?

Do other symptoms ever accompany the hives? If so, describe them.

Has the child recently received an inoculation of any kind?

Has the child recently started a course of new drugs, nose drops, sprays, tonics, laxatives, vitamins, cold tablets or other medication?

Has the child had any recent problems related to teeth, the intestinal tract, the urinary tract, fungal infections, appendicitis or tonsils?

Have you recently made any changes in your household cleaning or personal products such as soaps, detergents, bleaches and fabric softeners, shampoos, cosmetics, hair sprays, bath powders, dyes, mouthwashes, nail polish, toothpaste, and so on?

Have you recently brought any new or unusual items into the house such as furniture, drapes, chemicals? Have you painted your house lately?

Does the child tend to develop hives after touching cold objects such as snow or ice cubes?

Do hot or cold showers affect the child's condition?

Does any particular type of insect infest your home or immediate environment? Does the child experience allergic reactions to any type of insect bite?

Do the hives appear after a period of physical exertion and exercise?

Have you recently brought a pet into the house? Are there animals of any kind in the home environment? What are they?

Have you and/or the child recently visited new places? Have you recently moved your residence?

This list represents only a partial sampling of the questions an allergist might ask during an initial evaluation session *and* which you as parent should be prepared, as best you can, to answer thoroughly. The point must be made again that your doctor, even armed with answers to all the questions he may ask, can only diagnose the cause of acute hives in *less* than 30 percent of cases, while the cause of chronic hives can be diagnosed in less than *10* to *20* percent of cases. Not very happy statistics. But before you close this book and walk away, you should know that even if the cause of the hives ultimately eludes everyone, parents, physician and patient alike, the chances of medically *controlling* them remains very, very good.

Factors That Trigger Hives

If I tried to write down all the possible causes of hives, hundreds of pages would soon be filled with lists of foods, chemical agents, medical conditions, insects, and virtually every kind of pharmacologic agent in use today. The subject is vastly complex and extremely confusing. Still, an attempt must be made. The sections that follow, though certainly not inclusive of all the substances and situations that may cause hives, is complete enough to give you some idea of what to stay away from as well as where the major points of danger lie.

Drugs   Hives can develop owing to an allergic drug reaction or drug intolerance (see page 183). A sampling of medicines that can cause such trouble include:

> any antibiotics
> aspirin
> barbiturates
> codeine
> insulin
> iodides
> penicillin
> sulfa drugs
> tetanus antitoxin (horse serum)

Drugs of any type can cause hives. Discuss all medications with your physician to decide if you should continue to use them or if substitute drugs can be used. In the pediatric population, penicillin and its derivatives are probably the most likely of all drugs to trigger acute hives. Next in line comes aspirin (acetylsalicylic acid), which is capable of causing both acute and chronic cases in many sensitive children. In fact, any child who is prone to hives should steer clear of aspirin entirely and take acetaminophen in its place. Acetaminophen is sold over the counter under many brand names; two of the more common preparations are Tylenol and Datril.

A similar negative reaction may be caused by azo dyes, especially tartrazine. This chemical dye can be either yellow, red or purple and is used in foods and in many medicinal drugs including antihistamines. Another common preservative, benzoic acid, is present in many foods and drugs and can cause hives. The list of possible hive-producing substances by no means stops here and includes just about *any* drug or chemical.

It is therefore vitally important that parents keep an accurate record of all medications taken by their child, both prescription and over-the-counter varieties. This is one area of the child's personal medical history an allergist will most likely spend a good deal of time discussing with you.

Infection The possible cause-and-effect relationship between chronic low-grade infections of the tonsils, adenoids, sinuses, teeth, gall bladder or urinary tract and the development of hives has been debated by allergists for many years, and the final answer has yet to be resolved. I myself recall having seen two or three chronic hive sufferers whose symptoms disappeared when an unsuspected infection was discovered and treated. While I can provide no clear-cut medical reason why infection should be capable of causing hives, I do believe that for a very small number of patients such a relationship exists. Cases of this sort, I would add, are extremely rare and certainly would account for only a tiny percent of urticarial episodes.

Infestation with parasites Parasitic infection is another possible but somewhat unusual cause of chronic hives. The presence of animals in the home, poor personal hygiene habits, or recent trips taken to exotic places are all subjects your allergist will probably bring up with you at the initial interview. It is not easy to detect the presence of parasites in a person's body under any circumstances, and repeated examinations of multiple fresh stool specimens may be necessary if parasites are suspected. Once a specific type of parasite has been found, appropriate treatment is available.

Foods and food additives Though it is not possible to collect accurate statistics on the number of children who actually suffer from food-related hives, we know that foods are a common cause of hives. Hives can be triggered either by the foods themselves or by the chemical additives in the foods. Several of the more common offending foods include dairy products, eggs, peanuts, nuts, citrus fruits, tomatoes and shellfish. To this list add the multitudinous number of chemical additives, now somewhere in the hundreds, used in the growing, freshening and preserving of the foods we consume every day. Some of the more important representatives of this group include the tartrazine food dyes, and preservatives such as sodium benzoate, sulfite or metabisulfite. Soy products, which have been used as substitutes for milk-based infant formulas, can also trigger hives. With the increased use of soy products in our diet, allergists have been discovering more people who are allergic to this food.

Three important points to note about food-induced hives:

Acute urticaria is likely to be triggered by seasonal or unusual foods such as fresh vegetables and fruit, shellfish or strawberries.

Chronic urticaria is likely to be triggered by foods which are part of the normal daily diet such as wheat, milk or eggs.

Although an outbreak of hives usually follows immediately after the offending foods have been eaten, occasionally as much as eighteen to twenty-four hours may elapse before the first lesions appear.

What to do? While it is, of course, not always possible to pinpoint which ingested substances are responsible for hives, the use of a food diary will help. In this written record, *all* the foods your child eats each day must be carefully recorded. The list should cover snacks, school lunches, and "extracurricular" eating of any kind, including forbidden sweets. Useful as well is an elimination diet wherein specific foods and food groups are removed from the child's menu and any reaction to this change of diet is observed and recorded. As an example, if you suspect that your child's hives are triggered by milk, you can eliminate *all* dairy products from her diet for seven to ten days, note how much, if at all, the hives have improved. There is a further discussion of foods and food allergies in general in the chapter on food allergies. There is also a listing of foods that may cause hives starting on page 170.

Insect stings and bites   Before you can become allergic to a specific insect, you must be stung at least once by this creature in order to become sensitized. Though insect-induced hives are most often triggered by attacks from members of the order Hymenoptera—bees, wasps, hornets and yellow jackets—several other flying and crawling creatures can be responsible as well.

Papular urticaria, a hivelike eruption found primarily on the lower extremities, is caused by bites from bedbugs, fleas and mites. These lesions are usually more persistent than typical hives, smaller in appearance, and quite itchy.

In a child who has been sensitized to a specific caterpillar, contact with this wiggly creature will cause a linear-appearing itchy skin rash to develop. In the Northeast the gypsy moth caterpillar is especially likely to cause this problem; the rash is known as caterpillar dermatitis. Children who touch the gypsy moth caterpillar should immediately wash those parts of their bodies that have been in contact with the creature.

Occasionally, fly and mosquito stings can trigger hives. For further specifics on insect sting reactions see the following chapter.

Inhalants   Occasionally reports are heard in an allergist's office of hives being triggered by inhalants such as dander or pollen. If such a relationship can be firmly documented, then immunotherapy may be one method of helping the situation. From my experience, inhalant-caused hives are extremely unusual.

Physical agents   A wide variety of physical agents and conditions can produce an urticarial response. The following are the most common.

Sometimes called skin writing, *dermatographism* is an acute sensitivity of the skin to the force of friction. One of the most common types of physical urticaria, it takes the form of hivelike lesions that appear over any area that has recently been scraped or rubbed. The response can be easily elicited in sensitive children by running the blunt tip of a pen or pencil along the arms or legs; in a relatively short time a raised, reddened, occasionally itchy linear eruption will appear where the skin was stroked.

For some children, it also turns out, dermatographism can be a source of enormous pride and delight. Such youngsters have a great deal of fun allowing friends to draw pictures on their legs or to play tic-tac-toe across their forearms, making them the center of envy and attention. Perhaps this transformation of a liability into an asset is a blessing for the child too, for dermatographism is a permanent, lifetime phenomenon—nothing more, really, than a manifestation of highly sensitive skin.

Hives caused by *sudden exposure to cold temperatures* (cold urticaria)—e.g., running into the ocean, going from a warm house into the cold winter air—can be a potentially serious problem, triggering unpleasant symptoms such as headache, wheezing and on rare occasions severe breathing difficulties. A fifteen-year-old patient of mine named Jim once went for a swim in an icy mountain pond. Almost from the moment he entered the water his skin began to break out in hives from head to foot, and within a few minutes his breathing had became labored. Fortunately, there was an emergency room ten minutes away, and after an injection of epinephrine Jim's rash and wheezing subsided. Such a reaction is rare, it must be pointed out, and usually symptoms remain local, i.e., hives develop on the face and ungloved hands of a person taking a walk on a cold, windy day; an itchy rash appears on the hands when handling an ice cube. Typically, the symptoms of cold urticaria develop after exposure to the cold has taken place and the body is beginning to warm up. Jim's situation is somewhat unusual; however, it certainly is potentially dangerous for anyone who has this condition to jump into the ocean or dive into a pool!

The intensity of the symptoms that develop after exposure to a cold challenge will depend on the size of the body area chilled. For example, whenever Jane goes for a walk on a cold, wintry day, hives appear only on her face and hands (if she is not wearing gloves). Jim, on the other hand, rapidly developed generalized hives and breathing difficulties when his entire body was submerged in the pool. In either case there is no completely effective treatment, though the following measures may be taken to lessen the symptoms.

During the cold months of the year, cover the child's body as fully as possible whenever he ventures outdoors. This means gloves, hats, mufflers, the works.

In the summertime, make sure the child enters the ocean or swimming pool s-l-o-w-l-y. Diving is, of course, out of the question, as are any of the sudden immersion methods (such as pushing) that children and teenagers so enjoy. Let the child get acclimated to the water gradually, by degrees, especially when about to enter deep or potentially dangerous areas such as those found in a lake or ocean.

The antihistamine Periactin (cyproheptadine) is usually effective in blocking the effects of cold urticaria. It is only useful, however, when administered *before* exposure.

If you suspect that your child is suffering from cold urticaria, test your hunch by performing the "ice cube test." Place an ice cube directly on the child's forearm. Leave it there for five minutes, then take it away and examine the contact area. If as the area rewarms, a red, raised, itchy wheal appears on the spot in the exact shape of the ice cube, this is a positive response. This proves that cold urticaria is present.

Another form of urticaria is called *cholinergic urticaria.* This condition develops as a response to emotional stress, vigorous physical exertion, or heat exposure. The rash consists of many very small (less than one-eighth inch) raised wheals which are all intensely itchy.

Still another temperature-related rash is so-called *localized heat urticaria.* As its name suggests, it takes place on skin surfaces that are locally heated by a sun lamp, a flame, whatever. Relatively few cases have ever been recorded of this disorder, and I personally have never seen one.

In certain susceptible people, sunlight has the potential of producing a localized skin response called *solar urticaria.* This rash appears as hives on areas of the body frequently and directly exposed to the sun. Ordinarily seen in tropical or desert climates, it is by no means geographically limited and is occasionally reported in colder parts of this country, especially during the summer months. Solar urticaria is relatively unusual.

An unusual form of hives called *vibratory angioedema* is produced by skin contact with a rapidly shaking object, especially a mechanical object such as a throttle or the handle of a running lawn mower. The condition is rare and invariably inherited. Symptoms consist of hives, redness and localized swelling of the skin following stimulation of the contact area. The condition is usually noticed early in childhood and tends to persist throughout one's life. While it is rarely cause for serious concern, there is no specific cure for vibratory angioedema other than avoidance of contact with vibratory stimuli.

Typically *pressure urticaria and angioedema* results from a response, ordinarily a delayed response, to persistent pressure applied to various parts of the body. Tight clothing, belts, boots, bra straps, elastic on socks, a tight grip on a tennis racket, sitting in the same position for hours, any prolonged pressure can provoke it. Its identifying rash consists of itchy deep red wheals which appear up to four to six hours after the pressure stimulation has ceased.

Another unusual form of hives, *aquagenic urticaria,* is produced by skin contact with hot or cold water. Its characteristic rash has the same appearance as that caused by cholinergic urticaria, which is identified by its extremely small, red, extraordinarily itchy wheals. Very little is understood about this condition at the present time. As far as we know, it involves only a tiny percent of people who develop hives.

In the case of *exercise-induced urticaria,* hives or angioedema appear after a period of strenuous physical activity. While such outbreaks are usually mild, a particularly severe form does exist called exercise-induced anaphylaxis. I witnessed one such case several years ago. A teenage jogger taking his daily run suddenly developed severe wheezing along with an outbreak of hives. Gripped with an agonizing inability to catch his breath, the boy had to be rushed to a hospital where emergency measures with oxygen and epinephrine revived him. As with several of the other unusual varieties of urticaria mentioned, this condition is extremely rare.

Miscellaneous causes of hives A number of common and unusual urticarial conditions exist that do not fit into any of the categories mentioned so far.

Urticaria pigmentosa is a rather uncommon condition which consists of localized, slightly raised pigmented lesions. These areas are collections of mast cells under the skin. (Mast cells, you will recall, are white blood cells containing large amounts of histamine, the primary cause of hive formation.) If these areas are stroked or rubbed, histamine will be released from the cells and local hive formation will occur. Urticaria pigmentosa generally appears during the early childhood years and quite often vanishes when a youngster reaches puberty.

Hives may also appear as symptoms of other diseases. Ailments involving the collagen-vascular system (the connective and blood vessel systems) may produce chronic hives as early symptoms of an underlying condition. In fact, chronic generalized urticaria may on a rare occasion be an early symptom of a systemic disease such as rheumatoid arthritis, systemic lupus erythematosis, endocrine problems (especially hyperthyroidism), Hodgkin's disease or cancer of the colon. The point must be stressed, however, that these cases are extremely unusual; I have personally never seen a case in this category.

While anxiety-producing problems with family, friends, school, and so on can sometimes aggravate an existing urticarial condition, hives occurring *solely* on the basis of emotional problems are not very common. Let me also add that when a child's personal history is taken at the allergist's office, questions regarding the relationship between hives and the child's emotional state will inevitably be asked. Family members should be on guard against holding back critical information in this area out of fear of appearing inadequate or from worry of putting their child in a bad light. Remember, the doctor's interest is not in judging you or your child, only in eliminating the symptoms.

Hereditary angioedema (HAE) is caused by the absence or improper functioning of a specific enzyme of the complement system (known technically as Cl-esterase inhibitor) and is clinically characterized by recurring attacks of painful angioedema typically involving the skin and mucous membranes of the upper respiratory system and gastrointestinal tracts. These attacks in some patients may be triggered by mild physical trauma such as bumping into a wall or door. If your child has repeated complaints of abdominal pain and suffers from frequent swelling of the face and extremities, these symptoms should make you suspicious enough to contact your physician. The condition can be diagnosed by means of specific blood tests. Hereditary angioedema is a disease not to be taken lightly. When swelling involves the upper airways, the larynx can become blocked; death from suffocation has been reported in approximately 10 to 20 percent of HAE patients. Fortunately, laryngeal swelling usually takes several hours to develop, so that when and if respiratory involvement is discovered, HAE sufferers can usually get themselves to a physician or an emergency room before the attack becomes too severe. Hereditary angioedema, rare as it is, can definitely be *a life-threatening disease* and should be kept under strict medical supervision. Specific drug therapy is available today to control the condition.

A diagnosis of *idiopathic urticaria,* or idiopathic angioedema is the medical way of saying that we simply do not know what specific factors are causing the problem. This is the ultimate diagnosis in 50 to 70 percent of acute urticarial cases and 80 to 90 percent of chronic urticaria and angioedema cases.

Diagnostic Testing for Hives

In theory there is no limit to the number of diagnostic tests that can be ordered for a child with hives. In addition to blood samples, stool examinations and X-ray studies, consultations with a wide variety of specialists may be recommended. I do not advocate this zealous approach. I feel that after obtaining a detailed personal history and performing a thorough physical examination, a few basic screening tests are all that is needed to make a preliminary diagnosis and suggest a course of treatment. The first lab tests I generally order include:

a complete blood count (CBC) (see page 22)
a urinanalysis
an erythrocyte sedimentation rate determination test, used as a general
    screening test for infection or inflammation in the body.

If information is revealed in the child's personal history that suggests a specific cause for her hives, a number of other tests may possibly be ordered to confirm or disprove these suspicions. Such tests run the gamut from highly specific enzyme analysis to challenge tests using particular foods or other allergens. Your physician will suggest the tests which are most appropriate.

When the laboratory evaluation has been completed, and if the tests fail to show anything unusual, a diagnosis of idiopathic urticaria, either acute or chronic, will then be justified. Attention must next be focused on treatment.

Treatment of Hives and Angioedema

Environmental Control and Elimination Procedures

It is obvious that if the underlying cause of hives can be identified—foods, animals, chemicals, medicines or whatever—removal of these substances from the patient's environment will ordinarily cure the condition. While it is not always easy to determine the cause of hives, once the discovery has been made avoidance is the best way to clear up the condition.

A few general recommendations can be made:

1. Avoid giving your child any aspirin-containing preparations; use acetaminophen as a substitute.

2. Read food labels carefully and keep away from preservatives such as benzoates and members of the sulfite family. Do not use foods or medicines containing tartrazine dyes, especially FD&C Yellow No. 5.

3. If a pet dog or cat has proven to be the culprit causing the hives, then contact with the animal must be avoided.

4. For some of the more unusual types of physical stimuli (hot, cold, pressure, exertion) that may trigger the hives, the obvious recommendation is to avoid the situation that may bring on the symptoms.

Useful Medications for Hives

Antihistamines These drugs represent the first line of defense against symptoms of recurring urticaria; for the majority of patients, one or a combination of antihistamines will often be all the medication needed. As is commonly the case with antihistamines, however, it may take several tries on the doctor's part before the most effective antihistamine is discovered. While there are many antihistamines to choose from, it has been my clinical experience that hydroxyzine, marketed as Atarax or Vistaril, is the most effective for hives. I gradually increase the dose of this drug until the hives have disappeared completely for seven to ten days and then slowly lower the dose over a two- to four-week period. At the end of this time the hives have usually disappeared, and in approximately 80 to 90 percent of cases they do not return. Other antihistamines such as diphenhydramine (marketed as Benadryl) and cyproheptadine (marketed as Periactin) may be substituted for hydroxyzine if it cannot be tolerated or if it does not work. (For detailed information on antihistamines, see the chapter on asthma.)

Epinephrine (Adrenalin) For sudden episodes of severe, generalized hives or angioedema, treatment with epinephrine by injection usually brings rapid relief, though of a relatively short duration. This treatment can then be followed by a long-acting form of epinephrine called Sus-Phrine, which is effective for four to eight hours.

Metaproterenol and Terbutaline   Metaproterenol, marketed as either Alupent or Metaprel, and terbutaline, marketed as Bricanyl or Brethine, are occasionally prescribed for hives in combination with an antihistamine. Such combinations are sometimes more effective than the antihistamine alone.

Corticosteroids   Corticosteroids, when given in an appropriate dose, will successfully control almost all difficult cases of hives and angioedema. Because of their potentially dangerous side effects, however, these powerful preparations should be reserved for instances in which all other medications prove ineffective.

Regarding the dose, enough steroid medication should be given so that the hives are suppressed. The duration of treatment should be for the shortest possible time necessary to bring the symptoms under control. When the patient has been free of hives for three to four days, the dose can be decreased over the next four to six days. If steroids are abruptly discontinued, sometimes the hives will rebound in a more severe form; this is the reason for tapering the dose.

Last Thoughts

The ultimate outcome of urticaria and angioedema treatment depends on the underlying cause. Most acute cases are mild and self-limited; they appear and vanish without causing much difficulty. Soothing lotions such as calamine help in these situations, as do applications of wet baking soda or oatmeal. Avoid, however, Caladryl, a calamine lotion containing Benadryl that is often used to provide symptomatic relief for patients with hives. Benadryl alone is an excellent antihistamine when taken by mouth, but when used topically it can sensitize the skin and may cause a contact dermatitis. Anyone suffering with hives certainly doesn't need a second skin condition to worry about! Often nothing more elaborate than an over-the-counter cortisone ointment will do the trick. Whatever physical causes are the underlying trigger of this disorder, avoidance of the offending stimuli should control the symptoms. On the other hand, if urticaria is due to an underlying systemic disease, the outcome will naturally depend on the nature of the disease and the effectiveness of its treatment.

Finally, parents should be aware that chronic urticaria has a highly variable course: the symptoms may be present for several months or for many years. Periodic recurrences are not uncommon, though they are by no means guaranteed. In most cases this ailment is highly exasperating, at times causing itching so intense that patients feel like jumping out of their skins. Fortunately, except when associated with hereditary angioedema or with a malignant disease, urticaria is rarely life threatening and can usually be kept well controlled.

Questions and Answers on Hives and Angioedema

Should I be concerned if my child gets an occasional hive?

The appearance of one or two hives now and then is nothing to worry about. If the lesions are present for a short while and then clear up without medication, I would certainly not recommend consulting a professional. If, however, the hives are numerous, if they return frequently, and if they last for more than a day or so at a time, it would then be appropriate to discuss the situation with a physician.

Can hives be contagious?

The answer is a very definite no. You cannot "catch" hives by being in contact with someone who has them, just as you cannot catch asthma, angioedema and most other allergic ailments.

Are allergy injections appropriate for the treatment of hives?

It is theoretically possible for a child to develop hives as a result of a seasonal pollen sensitivity. In such an instance an argument could be made for the use of immunotherapy. Let me add, however, that in my many years of practice I have never seen such a case.

What role, if any, does climate or seasonal change play in chronic urticaria?

For most urticaria sufferers the changing seasons and variations in daily climate play little or no role in their condition. For those few children whose hives are triggered by winter weather (cold urticaria) or exposure to the sun (solar urticaria), a relationship obviously exists between the ailment and the seasons of the year. For these children appropriate precautions are always in order—wearing gloves and mufflers in cold weather, using sun screens out of doors.

Insect Sting Allergies

Andy, an active, outgoing six-year-old, was playing in the schoolyard one day during recess. Picking up a rock, he felt a sharp stinging sensation in his right hand. Quickly turning pale and becoming very anxious, he was taken to the school nurse, who cleaned what had become a large swelling on his wrist. Within a few minutes Andy seemed to be comfortable and was sent back to class. Five minutes later he returned to the nurse's office, complaining this time of chest pains; he was again very pale and quite uneasy. The school contacted his mother and she called Andy's doctor. By this time Andy was clearly in severe discomfort and a rescue squad was sent to transport him to the local hospital. There he was met by his pediatrician.

In the hospital, Andy was treated for what appeared to be a generalized reaction to an insect sting. Within an hour he was fine and ready to be discharged. The pediatrician's initial impression was that Andy had not reacted allergically to the sting but had experienced a fright response from the pain. The child was referred to my office to answer a number of his parents' questions. Was Andy really allergic to insect stings, and if so, what could be done about it? What medicines should the family keep at home and in school to cope with the problem? What would happen if Andy was stung again? Could such a reaction be triggered by fear alone? Could such a sting be fatal?

These are only some of the many questions asked thousands of times each year by parents of children who are allergic to insect stings. I want to review with you the current state of our knowledge regarding this frightening and often misunderstood condition, and then I will tell you how to cope with this situation.

The first fatality formally attributed to a wasp sting occurred in Egypt in 2641 B.C. The illustrious victim, according to temple hieroglyphics, was none other than the pharaoh himself, a ruler named Menes. Throughout unrecorded and recorded history stinging insects have regularly plagued humanity, though no one knows exactly how many of us are actually attacked each year by members of the more dangerous varieties, especially the Hymenoptera order of insects, whose ranks include bees, wasps, yellow jackets, hornets and the "fire ant." The multitude of people annually attacked by these aggressive creatures is in the millions, of course, but, happily, estimates from studies suggest that 99.5 percent of victims have nothing more serious to worry about than a bit of temporary discomfort.

For our purposes there remains the one-half of 1 percent to consider, and for these people the situation may be hazardous and even life-threatening— on the average forty to sixty reported deaths each year are *directly* attributed to insect sting reactions. Fortunately for young people, the vast majority of these fatalities occur in adults, and in fact it is very unusual for a child to die from a sting of any kind, even if the child is highly allergic. Still, caution is the watchword, especially if you know for certain that your child is vulnerable. First, let's identify the cast of villains.

The Order Hymenoptera

Within this biological group the female alone is capable of delivering a sting. We know this for certain because only the female possesses a stinger. Important among the Hymenoptera are the following families of insects:

Apidae The principal here is the honeybee, a small, hairy insect decorated with yellow or tan stripes. Honeybees live in man-made hives or in hives constructed in trees, stumps and caves. As a rule, honeybees are relatively unaggressive creatures; most stings occur when bees are stepped on or when their hives are menaced.

Unfortunately for the bee, its stinger and its intestines are attached to one another. Since the bee inevitably eviscerates itself when trying to pull its barbed stinger free from the sting site, the delivery of its sting is tantamount to suicide. (Honeybees are the only members of the order Hymenoptera with barbed stingers.) Thus a child can be stung only once by the same bee, and anyone who shows signs of several bee stings has, ipso facto, been stung by several different attackers. Another point: if your child has been stung and the stinger is visible and protruding, remember that significant amounts of venom are still

Honeybee

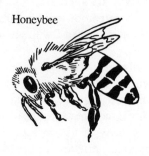

present in the sac attached to the stinger. Grabbing the stinger as if it were a splinter and moving it around will only end up forcing more venom into the unfortunate victim. The best thing to do under these circumstances is to flick the stinger off with the thumb and forefinger, as quickly and as smoothly as possible.

Bombidae The most important member in this group is the bumblebee. This large, noisy, ponderous creature covered with yellow and black bands is almost never guilty of stinging anyone. It does have the necessary apparatus to sting, but it takes enormous aggressiveness on the part of any adult or child to force an attack. In general, despite their frightening appearance bumblebees are not insects to worry about.

Vespidae In this group we find some of nature's most insistent aggressors: yellow jackets, hornets and wasps.

Of all insects, yellow jackets are most frequently the cause of allergic sting reactions, perhaps because they are particularly predisposed to attack humans. Aggressive by nature, they become particularly pugnacious late in the summer when living space in the hives gets overcrowded. Their nests are usually constructed in the ground or near decaying trees, and they can be seen swarming around open garbage cans or trash baskets. To date, fifteen species of yellow jackets have been identified in this country, and there is scarcely an area of the United States where they do not breed.

Hornets Though hornets look somewhat like yellow jackets with their yellow stripes and short-waisted bodies, they are generally larger and less hairy. Similarly aggressive, they build aboveground nests that can be easily identified by their typical football-shaped appearance and by their gray, paper-like outer walls, which the hornets manufacture themselves from the masticated fiber of plants and wood. Unlike the honeybee—and like their cousins, the wasps and yellow jackets—a hornet has an unbarbed stinger. This means it can sting, remove its stinger safely, and sting again without suffering any ill effect. This fact, added to its nervous, irascible disposition, makes the hornet a creature well worth avoiding.

Wasps These creatures have a narrow, hairless body characterized by a tapered waist. Wasps build their small, open, honeycombed nests in trees,

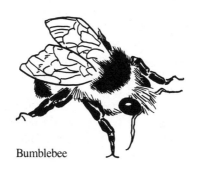

Bumblebee

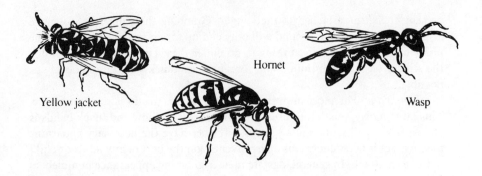

shrubs and especially the eaves of houses. Somewhat less aggressive than yellow jackets and hornets, wasps nonetheless deliver a painful sting when riled.

Clinical Reactions to Insect Stings

What reactions might you expect following the sting of a member of the Hymenoptera order? In general, there are three types: local, generalized multi-organ system response, and unusual.

Local reactions A local reaction is the type of response a *non*allergic individual develops when stung. It consists of a sharp, burning sensation at the site of the sting, caused by toxic substances contained in the insect's venom. Within five to fifteen minutes, local swelling and redness will appear, and all signs of the reaction usually vanish within twelve to twenty-four hours. At times a local reaction can also involve a large area of the body: a hand, an entire arm or even the whole face. The important thing to remember when such a thing occurs is that this response, no matter how dramatic and uncomfortable it may be, is in no way life threatening.

Generalized multi-organ system response If a child is stung on the arm, and if hives and breathing difficulties soon develop, that child is experiencing what is known as an anaphylactic reaction. The crucial thing to observe is whether or not the developing symptoms involve areas of the body distant from the sting site. If that is the situation, you can be certain that an allergic response is taking place. A generalized or constitutional reaction requires *prompt medical treatment.* Remember, if your child is stung on the finger and her face becomes swollen—get to a doctor!

Observe also that a generalized reaction, or for that matter any kind of allergic response to an insect sting, can occur *only* after a person has been sensitized to the venom of that insect. In other words, to develop an allergic sensitivity to an insect your child must have been stung by the same creature or a related family member at least once and possibly many times at some earlier date. The intensity of the response that follows can range from a mild outbreak of hives to a severe systemic reaction causing a sudden drop of blood pressure, generalized swelling, a tight sensation in the throat, and difficulty breathing. Death can ultimately result if the condition is not treated promptly.

Allergic reactions can begin within minutes after the sting or several hours after the attack. The symptoms can be mild, characterized by skin eruptions, general redness and itching, hives and angioedema (swelling of the lips, nose and ears). Or they may be far more serious, consisting of some or all of the following:

> involvement of the airways. Symptoms may include tightness in the chest, shortness of breath, hoarse voice (which comes from swelling of the larynx and throat) and wheezing
>
> a severe drop in blood pressure (hypotension) with accompanying confusion, paleness and possible loss of consciousness
>
> intestinal symptoms such as nausea, vomiting and pain

In its most severe form, an anaphylactic reaction to a sting can be fatal. As mentioned earlier, however, it is extremely rare for children to die from such causes.

Generalized toxic reactions are produced not by an allergy but by a reaction to the poisonous substances in the insect's venom. This type of reaction occurs only after someone has received many, many stings within a short period of time. The accumulated toxins contained in the venom are thought to be responsible for the following symptoms:

> headache
> dizziness
> fever
> gastrointestinal complaints: nausea, vomiting, pain, diarrhea
> convulsions

Unusual or atypical reactions   These reactions, not caused by an allergic reaction, are almost always delayed in their onset. The parts of the body involved are almost always the vascular and nervous systems. Responses include clotting defects in the blood, bloody diarrhea, neuritis and partial paralysis. Less common are fever, joint aches and pains, enlargement and tenderness of the lymph nodes, hives and angioedema. When these somewhat mysterious symptoms do occur, they may last only a day or so, or they may continue for several weeks. In general, these reactions are quite rare.

Diagnosing Allergic Insect Sting Reactions

How does your doctor go about determining whether or not your child has actually had an allergic sting reaction? There are several ways.

As I have stressed in preceding chapters, the more complete the presentation of the child's personal medical history at the time of the initial visit, the easier it will be for an allergist to piece together the evidence and make a specific diagnosis. This rule holds particularly true for insect stings. Why? Referral to an allergist for an insect sensitivity usually takes place days to weeks after the reaction to the sting has subsided. A physical examination will be given, of course, but since the symptoms have disappeared there is not a lot to be learned from this avenue of investigation. The personal history therefore emerges as the physician's strongest—if not *only*—link to the event, and for this reason the doctor must be provided with a very complete history. Often, of course, a child will realize that she has been stung only after the insect has flown away, so that visual identification of the offender is generally not possible. Nevertheless, information regarding the overall circumstances of the episode is immensely helpful. Such information may include any of the following facts:

Where was the child when the sting occurred? Indoors? Outdoors? In the woods? In a flower garden? In a barn or on a picnic? Inside the house?

Was there any evidence of a hive or nest nearby? If so, where was it located? Describe it in detail. Was there specific vegetation close by, such as rotting logs or an orchard in bloom?

Were there any garbage bags or open trash receptacles in the vicinity?

Was the child stung more than once?

Was a stinger found in the wound? Did you or the child attempt to remove it, and if so, how?

What were the child's immediate symptoms? How long did it take for these symptoms to appear after the sting? Describe the progress and development of the symptoms in detail.

How long did the symptoms last?

After a patient's history has been obtained, several laboratory tests may be in order. Standard testing procedures for insect stings include direct skin test methods and blood tests.

Skin Tests

Direct skin tests Direct skin tests are certainly the method of choice for the evaluation of aeroallergen (pollen) sensitivity; however, with Hymenoptera sensitivity this may not be the case. Direct skin tests for most insect allergy patients are an excellent method of establishing a diagnosis. For a small percentage of venom sensitive children it may be necessary to perform a RAST test to confirm the diagnosis.

From a practical point of view it is necessary to wait at least two weeks after a suspected reaction has occurred before direct tests can be done. The testing will proceed in the usual manner of skin tests, beginning with an extremely diluted specific venom sample. The starting test dose will be 1/200,000th to 1/2,000,000th of the amount contained in a single sting. If the patient does not react to these low concentrations they will be gradually increased, the strongest dose is equal to 1/50th the strength of a usual sting. The testing procedure involves the use of both the prick/puncture and intracutaneous techniques (see pages 26–28 for details of these procedures).

Direct skin tests are highly accurate in confirming an allergic sensitivity to a specific insect. The main drawback of skin tests is that they are obviously performed directly on the patient. This situation creates the possibility of triggering a generalized reaction. In practice, such reactions are extremely rare, and so far I have never encountered this problem.

Blood Tests

Some physicians feel that the RAST test is a highly accurate method of testing for insect sting allergy. One drawback is the 15 to 20 percent of false negative tests obtained by the RAST technique. A false negative test is one that fails to show a positive reaction in someone who is truly allergic to a member of the Hymenoptera. A possible explanation for this response is felt to be an insufficient amount of IgE antibody circulating in the bloodstream. The direct skin test looks for IgE antibody which has already attached itself to the tissue mast cells.

One significant advantage of RAST over direct testing is that the patient doesn't run a risk of reacting to the RAST test. For the individual who had a severe anaphylactic reaction to the insect sting, the RAST test would probably be my first choice as a diagnostic procedure.

Another kind of blood test, not generally available and performed only in a few specialized research centers around the country, is the leukocyte histamine release procedure. Here a measurement is taken of the amount of histamine released by a patient's white blood cells when stimulated by a specific insect venom. This study is ordinarily used to confirm a questionable direct or RAST test result.

RAST testing appears to be a good method of checking on the effectiveness of an immunotherapy program. Your allergist may periodically perform this test to check how well your child is responding to this treatment.

Whole Body Extracts: A Brief Note of Warning

Until 1979 the only material available for the diagnosis and treatment of Hymenoptera sensitivity was known as whole body extract. This preparation was produced by pulverizing an insect, processing its remains, and producing a mixture composed of the entire body. The resulting whole body extract was then used to test and treat patients with Hymenoptera sensitivity. As you can imagine, there was much material in this final product that was without therapeutic value of any kind. In a number of clinical studies it was proven that the use of whole body insect extract for both testing and treatment was ineffective and should be discontinued.

So if your child is currently being treated with whole body extracts, you should know that this procedure is decidedly out-of-date. In my opinion, your child should be retested for insect sensitivities using specific Hymenoptera venoms. If positive results are obtained, consideration should then be given to starting treatment with specific venom immunotherapy.

Treatment for Insect Sting Allergies

There are three principal approaches to the treatment of insect sting allergies: preventive methods of avoiding insect stings, symptomatic medications for acute sting reactions, and immunotherapy.

Prevention of Stings

Of all allergic conditions, insect sting reactions may be the easiest to avoid. The process is simple: no contact; no sting; no reaction. Toward this aim the following suggestions are offered. No doubt you will have methods of your own to add to the list:

> The risk of being stung peaks in the late summer and early fall when Hymenoptera nests are particularly crowded and active.

> Have your child avoid areas where insects feed: orchards in bloom, clover fields, flower gardens, garbage disposal sites, and picnic grounds.

> Do not let your child wear perfumes, colognes, scented deodorants and hair sprays.

> Make sure your child avoids playing or working in the yard near bushes, trees, stumps or any area where insect nests are usually found.

> If there is a nest on your property, have it removed by a professional. Exterminators are the obvious choice for this task; you might also consider calling a local beekeeper if the offending nest is a beehive or a swarm of bees.

> Keep the windows of your car closed both when parked and when driving. Check the inside of an automobile for insects before getting in.

Always have your child wear shoes when playing outdoors. Walking barefoot on a lawn or in a field is an invitation to a sting.

Do not outfit your child with loose-fitting clothes. These may end up acting as a kind of net, entangling insects rather than protecting against them.

Always keep a can of insecticide in your home and car.

Do not dress your child in floral prints or highly colored clothes; these patterns are especially attractive to flying insects.

If your child has already experienced a severe reaction to an insect sting, he should wear some type of identification tag describing the condition. A Medic-Alert bracelet is excellent for this purpose. Parents are also well advised to keep an emergency insect sting kit on hand at all times. Prescriptions for these kits will be supplied by your physician.

Learn and continually review the steps that must be taken in times of a sting emergency. Talk these steps over with your doctor until you are certain you understand everything involved: forewarned is forearmed.

Medical Treatment for an Acute Sting

Treatment for an insect sting depends on the severity and nature of the sting itself. It is a question of degree.

A sting that does not cause an allergic reaction can be controlled by cleaning the area with alcohol and placing ice on the site to control swelling. If a stinger is protruding, flick it away with a knife blade or a fingernail. A standard home remedy for reducing pain is to mix baking soda with a small amount of water and apply it to the wound. All visible traces of the sting should be gone within a day or two.

For any generalized allergic reaction, the most effective medication is epinephrine (Adrenalin). If your child has had a generalized reaction to an insect sting, then epinephrine is available for self-administration either in an Ana-Kit or an EpiPen. The contents of an Ana-Kit include epinephrine in a prefilled syringe and several antihistamine tablets. The EpiPen is a disposable injection device containing a preloaded dose of epinephrine which automatically discharges when pressed firmly against the skin. Your doctor will demonstrate the proper technique for giving Adrenalin with either the Ana-Kit or EpiPen.

Even if a sensitized child has been given an injection of epinephrine at the sting site, she should still be rushed to a hospital emergency room for observation. In most instances the only treatment will be an antihistamine given to

control local swelling that persists even after the epinephrine has been administered.

If the sting site becomes infected, it can easily be treated with appropriate
antibiotic therapy.

Immunotherapy

While venom immunotherapy has been proven to be 96 to 98 percent effective
in preventing generalized allergic reactions to insect stings, it should only be
given to individuals who meet *certain specific requirements.* (See page 42 for
detailed information on immunotherapy.) Exactly what these requirements are
has been defined and redefined during the past decade as allergists have accumulated more and more case histories and as new research has been evaluated. Generally speaking, the two following conditions are necessary before
venom immunotherapy should be recommended.

A documented history must exist of a generalized reaction to an insect
sting. The reaction must have involved either the respiratory and/or the
cardiovascular system and have been serious enough to cause a drop in blood
pressure (hypotension, fainting) or airway obstruction (swelling of the throat,
difficulty in breathing, wheezing).

Positive test results must be obtained either by direct skin tests or the
RAST technique. Negative test results combined with a positive medical history do *not* qualify a child as a candidate for immunotherapy.

When and if a positive history and confirming test results are obtained,
the next step is to begin the venom immunotherapy injections. The usual
schedule calls for weekly visits to the allergist for ten to fourteen weeks, then
one visit every other week for two doses. Finally, a maintenance schedule
consists of monthly visits. At the present time, maintenance programs which
extend the dosing period to once every six weeks or longer are being evaluated,
and the reports so far seem very promising.

Currently, several researchers are studying RAST-determined antibody
levels as a possible method of predicting when it will be safe to discontinue
immunotherapy. Hopefully, within the year or two we will be able to answer
the constantly repeated question "How much longer do I have to take these
shots?"

What side effects may occur from venom immunotherapy? Most patients
experience no discomfort of any kind. When a reaction does occur, it is almost
always localized, consisting of redness, swelling and some immediate or
delayed pain at the injection site. A word of caution: while anaphylaxis is an
extremely rare side effect of immunotherapy, isolated cases have been reported.
It is therefore important that your child wait in the physician's office for at
least twenty to thirty minutes after the injections have been given. Most

anaphylactic reactions, when they do take place, ordinarily occur within the first half hour after treatment.

Notes on Fire Ants and Other Insect Pests

The fire ant, which can both bite and sting, gets its name because its victims feel as though they have been "burned" after being attacked. This is a nonflying member of the Hymenoptera that is currently found only in the southern states. However, there is a growing concern that this pest may spread into most of the temperate areas of the country.

Fire ants are highly aggressive. They possess the unfortunate ability to both bite *and* sting, and they will assault humans and animals alike with fearless abandon. Reactions to their attacks range from a localized, painful burning sensation to generalized anaphylaxis. Characteristically, their sting produces a pustule that develops fully within twenty-four hours after the attack. If your doctor suspects such a reaction, appropriate testing methods are available, and venom therapy is usually quite effective against sensitivity to this unpleasant creature.

As an allergist I am also frequently asked if treatments exist to control "allergic" reactions caused by flies and mosquitoes. First, let me say that these insects do not sting, they *bite.* In order to sting, a creature must have a stinger capable of injecting venom; neither flies nor mosquitoes possess such an apparatus. Moreover, the reaction following their bites is almost always local and almost never allergic. True, some children develop a very large swelling from mosquito bites, but this response is not an allergic one.

There have been reports of anaphylactic reactions following the bites of bedbugs and kissing bugs. These small, blood-sucking creatures work their mischief while their victims sleep, and they can indeed trigger a serious response, though only on the rarest occasions. The best method of controlling them is avoidance: increased personal hygiene and regular changing and laundering of the bedding are both mandatory.

In recent years the northeastern states have also had a problem with gypsy moth caterpillars; rashes caused by them have been reported with increasing frequency both among children and adults. The use of insecticides, proper protective sprays in surrounding trees and avoidance of physical contact are all proven methods of protection against this pest. (See the section on insect stings and bites in the chapter on hives for more information on gypsy moth reactions, page 144.)

Finally, general recommendations for the treatment of insect bites include the use of topical steroid creams to decrease itching plus antihistamines such as Benadryl and Atarax for control of localized swelling. In the unlikely event that a generalized allergic reaction occurs, epinephrine is once again the best of all remedies. Unfortunately, at this time no forms of immunotherapy exist capable of controlling allergic reactions to insects outside the Hymenoptera.

Questions and Answers on Insect Sting Allergies

Is a child who has hay fever more likely to have an allergic reaction to an insect sting than a nonallergic child?

There is no evidence that I know of to indicate that a child with an allergic problem of *whatever* kind is more likely than a nonallergic child to develop insect sting sensitivities.

Is insect sting allergy inherited?

As far as we know, there is no indication of a hereditary pattern. If you or your parents, or your siblings, uncles and aunts for that matter, suffer from an insect sting allergy, you can rest assured that this in no way increases the chances of your own children developing such a problem.

Will the use of an insect repellent protect a child against the sting of a bee, wasp, hornet, yellow jacket or fire ant?

No. Repellent will sometimes keep flies, fleas and mosquitoes at bay. Against members of the Hymenoptera it is practically useless. Don't depend on it for that purpose.

How can you tell if a child is having an allergic reaction to an insect sting?

One simple method, as mentioned earlier, is to look for symptoms on the body distant from the sting site. For example, if a child is stung on the hand and she develops an itchy rash on her chest, she is having an allergic reaction. If she is stung on the ear and develops difficulty catching her breath, it's the same thing.

How soon after a person has been stung will an allergic reaction usually begin?

The answer depends on several factors. How allergic is the child? What part of the body was stung? Was the child stung more than once? While you will ordinarily be able to identify a generalized anaphylactic reaction within the first few minutes after the sting, several hours may pass before any sign of reaction begins with ordinary allergic symptoms. Certainly it would be extremely unusual if any allergic symptoms took more than a twenty-four-hour period to appear.

My daughter has been stung on two occasions by yellow jackets. The second time her entire arm swelled up twice its normal size. Should she be given immunotherapy for this reaction?

No, immunotherapy injections are not indicated for such local reactions regardless of their severity. Recommendations for treatment are made only if a child shows a generalized reaction with evidence of breathing difficulty, a drop in blood pressure or a loss of consciousness.

Food Allergies

An area of particular frustration for parents and allergists alike is the murky, unpredictable world of food allergies. If you listen to the many "experts" holding forth on radio and TV today or if you read certain pseudoscientific publications lining the pop bookshelves, you may already believe that food allergies are as common as headaches or that they produce a range of symptoms that run the gamut from anxiety to arthritis. We are told by these "experts" that children who are bothered by insomnia, who have discipline problems or trouble concentrating in class, are actually suffering from an allergy to some unnamed antigen in their morning cereal or to a chemical in their school lunch. Some physicians go so far as to say that they possess infallible diagnostic methods by which they can magically determine which foods are causing the troublesome symptoms and then clear the whole thing up tidily with appropriate diet therapy.

I only wish these claims were true and that it was possible to resolve such problems by merely regulating your child's menu. But the food allergy question is far more complicated and undefined than certain elements of the lay press would have you believe, and allergists are still groping for fundamental answers. In this chapter you will learn the crucial things that we *do* know about food allergies, and perhaps more importantly, you will find out what workable therapies exist to control them.

Food Allergy Versus Food Intolerance

While the actual incidence of food allergy among children is very difficult to determine, there are unquestionably fewer cases than some physicians and lay preachers would have us believe. Many reactions labeled allergic later turn out to stem from other causes. At this point, before things get too confused, let's define and explain our terms.

Food allergy reaction Allergic reactions to food develop *only* when an individual becomes sensitized to a particular food. This means that specific antibodies (IgE class proteins) have been produced which indicates that the child is now sensitized. Each time the youngster is given that food—egg, for example—an allergic reaction will take place, causing chemical mediators to be released into the bloodstream. These chemical mediators—histamine being the most familiar—then produce the spectrum of allergic symptoms. These symptoms may involve not only the intestinal tract where the food is digested (vomiting, diarrhea) but also the skin (hives, eczema) and the lungs (asthma). A person highly allergic to a food can have an anaphylactic reaction after eating a small amount of that food (see page 6 for a complete description of the allergic triggering process).

Food intolerance reaction   Clinically, a food intolerance is often mistaken for an allergic response. However, from a theoretical point of view the two are fundamentally different. A food intolerance reaction does not involve allergic sensitization; there is therefore no production of IgE antibodies within the bloodstream. Let's look at some of the prominent factors that trigger this response.

Food poisoning   This type of response occurs as a result of the direct action of either the food or an additive chemical. It does not involve an allergic or immune reaction. Symptoms occur because of toxins (poisons) released by bacteria or parasites that have contaminated the food.

Anaphylactoid reaction   Whenever there is a generalized release of chemical mediators in the body that is not caused by an allergic triggering response, we have what is known as an anaphylactoid reaction. This reaction produces generalized intestinal, respiratory and skin responses which by all outward signs appear to be the same as those typical of an anaphylactic reaction; yet, to stress the fact again, this response is *not* induced by allergic causes. Anaphylactoid reactions can occur after the ingestion of foods which contain large amounts of the chemical histamine, such as tuna fish, mackerel and Swiss cheese.

Metabolic food reaction   This response is triggered by food substances that have an adverse affect on a child's normal metabolism. Symptoms include diarrhea, cramps and bloating, all of which can occur within the first few weeks of an infant's life. As a rule, such reactions are experienced by individuals who are already weakened by malnutrition, disease or medicines that affect normal metabolic functions.

A good example of a metabolic food reaction is the inherited absence of an enzyme in the system called lactase, a substance necessary for the proper digestion of lactose. Children born with this condition cannot digest dairy products—lactose is the milk sugar found in most dairy products—and hence must be fed milk substitutes such as soy formula. Some population groups appear to be at greater risk than others. Among North American blacks, for instance, 70 to 80 percent suffer from bowel wall lactase deficiency, while 55 to 95 percent of Asians have the same problem. Contrast these figures with the low 5 to 20 percent incidence in North American Caucasians, or with the 3 percent incidence among Danish children. If a child has lactose intolerance, the condition will usually reveal itself early in life, sometimes during the first weeks. Parents of newborns should be on the alert for this problem, and should quickly seek a physician's advice if their child seems unable to tolerate a milk-based formula.

Recognizing the Symptoms of Food Allergy

If it is indeed so difficult to recognize and diagnose food allergies, what symptoms, if any, can be considered at least suggestive of an allergic food reaction?

From one standpoint the answer is that no single symptom or even pattern of symptoms offers foolproof evidence. In fact, the only way to properly diagnose a food allergy is by careful observation of *all* symptoms, even those which do not originate in the gastrointestinal tract. However, at the same time, the two systems where allergic symptoms caused by food sensitivity are most likely to occur are the gastrointestinal tract and the skin.

Gastrointestinal Symptoms

Any child who ingests a food to which he is allergic may develop immediate symptoms that can start with an itching sensation of the lips. This reaction is frequently followed by localized swelling of the lips, mouth and tongue; occasionally the swelling becomes so severe that it obstructs the breathing tubes and impairs breathing, creating a life-threatening situation. One young patient of mine had a reaction of this kind every time she ate cashew nuts. Another developed difficulty breathing whenever he ate eggs or lobster.

As we progress deeper into the gastrointestinal tract, the primary symptoms are cramping abdominal pain accompanied by nausea, vomiting and diarrhea. A list of the most common gastrointestinal reactions includes:

swelling of the tongue and throat
localized itching of the lips and mouth
difficulty in swallowing
nausea and vomiting
general abdominal pain and "stomachache"
diarrhea
itching of the anal area
bleeding from the small and large intestine (unusual)

Symptoms of the Skin

Though often difficult to pinpoint, food allergies are one of the principal causes of hives and angioedema among younger children. Eggs, dairy products and wheat are the main offenders here, though foods such as nuts, peanuts, shellfish, chocolate and berries may contribute as well. No part of the body is immune from food-induced hives or angioedema. Typical allergic responses of the skin include:

itching
redness and burning of the skin
hives and/or angioedema
atopic dermatitis

Other Areas Where Food-Allergic Symptoms May Appear

There are some children who develop coughing and wheezing as the result of food allergies. The incidence of asthma attacks triggered by a specific food sensitivity, however, is not very high, and when it does occur it is usually obvious which food is to blame. The most common offender in this instance is milk and other dairy products, followed by corn, peanuts and eggs.

An allergic food reaction may also trigger such classically allergic symptoms as sneezing, runny nose, tearing, red and swollen eyes, shortness of breath, rapid heartbeat, shock and collapse. These signs occur singly, or, on rare occasions, all at once, in which case a severe generalized allergic response is at work: anaphylaxis. A food reaction of this intensity is rare but when it occurs it is a *medical emergency* and requires a doctor's attention.

Finally, some physicians feel that a variety of symptoms such as hyperactivity, joint pains, bed wetting, insomnia, fatigue, migraine headaches, anxiety, muscular aches, depression, and arthritis are caused by food allergies. This notion is based on what I consider to be inadequate evidence, as many of the procedures used to document the "allergic" nature of these symptoms —and many of the methods employed to treat them—can at best be described as controversial. (A discussion of unproven diagnostic and therapeutic techniques in treating allergies will be found in the chapter "Parents Beware.")

Foods Most Likely to Trigger Allergic Reactions

This rather lengthy list begins with the first food for most of us: milk.

Cow's milk   Most infants who are not breast fed are initially fed with a formula derived from cow's milk. Since an infant's intestinal tract is still relatively immature, milk proteins can easily pass through the intestinal wall and react with cells of the immune system, thus getting an early start on allergic sensitization. Milk allergy, as a result, is one of the most frequent and early of all food problems. Its symptoms run the gamut from nasal congestion, to severe vomiting and chronic diarrhea, to allergic skin rashes such as atopic dermatitis and hives. It can be caused by dairy products of all kinds including cheese, ice cream, ice milk, yogurt and butter as well as foods containing milk solids, casein, caseinate and lactalbumin.

What to do about milk allergies? Eliminate milk and milk products from your child's diet. Fortunately there are a number of corporations you can write to for milk-free recipes and meal planners (see "Sources for Specific Diet Information," page 272). Better yet, most children who develop dairy allergies outgrow them after several years. In my experience the great majority of children who are allergic to cow's milk during the first one to two years of life come to tolerate it quite nicely by the time they are five to seven years old.

Cereal grains This very common food group is found in an almost limitless number of preparations we eat on a daily basis. The major representatives are wheat, corn, millet, rye, oats, barley and rice. Of the seven, wheat and corn are by far the most frequent and serious offenders. Allergic symptoms triggered by grain tend to involve the gastrointestinal tract, producing nausea, vomiting, abdominal pains and diarrhea, though symptoms such as rhinitis, asthma and hives can also occur.

One of the hazards of cereal allergies is that both wheat and corn are "hidden" in many common foods, especially corn in the form of cornstarch or corn sweeteners. Watch out for the following commercial food items, all of which contain one or both of these grains:

baked beans (corn)	candy bars (corn/wheat)
beer (corn)	chowders (corn/wheat)
chewing gum (corn)	gravy (wheat/corn)
corn oil	ice cream cones (corn/wheat)
glue on envelopes and stamps (corn)	lunch meats (wheat/corn)
ketchup (corn)	coffee substitute (wheat)
marshmallows (corn)	fried chicken (wheat)
mayonnaise (corn)	gluten flour (wheat)
popcorn	graham flour (wheat)
powdered sugar (corn)	hot dogs (wheat)
salad dressing (corn)	macaroni (wheat)
whiskey (corn)	spaghetti (wheat)

These hidden sources can in most instances be avoided by scrutinizing food labels and avoiding any products that contain the offending substances. If you have any questions, contact the manufacturers directly.

What about rye? Is it a good substitute for wheat bread? Because an all-rye bread won't rise, from 40 to 60 percent of all rye bread recipes call for wheat flour in addition to the rye. A 100 percent rye bread is available but hard to find. The best bet is the bakery shelves of a natural foods store, or better yet, your own home oven. (See the Appendix for listings of companies that can supply you with special wheat-free products.)

Citrus fruits   The citrus family includes oranges, tangerines, grapefruits, lemons, limes, kumquats and a few other fruits. Many children develop allergic intestinal symptoms from these foods, especially from orange juice. Contact dermatitis is a local inflammatory, irritative skin reaction that can occur after many substances, including foods, cosmetics and certain types of jewelry touch the skin. This type of response may develop around the mouth when a citrus food comes in contact with the area. Some youngsters can tolerate small amounts of citrus juices, especially if the juice is watered down and not consumed on a daily basis. Be aware that some forms of fruit punch or fruit drink such as grape or apple may contain citrus juices hidden in the mixture and are a potential source of trouble.

Chocolate   Of all the foods we have mentioned, chocolate is undoubtedly the least essential for children *and* the most difficult to prevent them from eating. A related member of this food family is the cola nut, and hence cola drinks such as Coke, Pepsi and Dr Pepper, to name a few favorites, should be eliminated from the diet of any child with a chocolate sensitivity.

The following substances infrequently cause allergic reactions:

apples or apple juice	plums
bananas	potatoes
barley	rice
beef	rye
beets	salt
carrots	soybean milk
grape juice	spring water
lamb	squash
lettuce	sweet potatoes
oats	tea
peaches	turkey
pears	

These substances *most often* cause allergic reactions:

chocolate	nuts
eggs	pork
fish	shellfish
fresh fruit, especially berries	tomato products
milk	

Evaluating Food Allergies

Your visit to an allergist will be especially productive if you come prepared to answer specific questions concerning your child's condition. Typical of a doctor's queries are the following:

What specific food-related symptoms have you observed? Describe in as much detail as you can the pattern of these symptoms.

When do symptoms occur in relation to meals?

How long do these symptoms last?

Have the allergic patterns changed since you first began to notice them? In what ways?

Does the child have any particular food cravings? Does she actively avoid certain foods? Which ones?

What treatment, if any, has been used to relieve the symptoms? How successful has it been?

Are you suspicious of a specific food or food group such as dairy products, egg-containing substances or citrus fruits? On what evidence is your suspicion based?

What foods does your child normally eat? Give sample breakfast, lunch and dinner menus. Information on the child's favorite foods, her snacking patterns, the amounts of food the child eats, will all be helpful.

For an infant, all facts regarding formula will be crucial. So will all recent changes in the diet and information on the child's general eating patterns, the sequence of new foods recently introduced to the diet and the kinds of vitamins being taken.

Are other members of the child's family allergic to any particular foods? Which ones? Is there allergy of any kind in your family? If so, describe it.

What is the child's general allergic history, if any? Is the child presently being treated for other allergic problems?

Describe your child's physical growth history. If possible, provide height and weight charts. These will be evaluated to determine if she is developing normally.

If your child vomits frequently, how soon after eating does the vomiting take place? Describe the appearance of the vomited material.

How often does the child have a bowel movement? Is the stool usually well formed or is it watery, hard, loose, bloody? Does it have any unusual odor?

This list is, of course, only a sampling of the many possible questions that will be reviewed in depth. The child's medical and allergic history is the allergist's single most effective diagnostic tool.

Following the taking of the history, a complete physical examination will be performed. The doctor will be looking for typical signs and symptoms of allergy such as skin rashes, dark circles under the eyes, nasal congestion and wheezing. In addition, the doctor will make a general assessment of your child's nutritional condition: how good is the muscle tone? Is the child over-weight or underweight?

Following this examination the allergist must then decide which tests, if any, are required to complete the evaluation. General screening procedures that may be called for include:

A serum IgE level test   IgE is the specific protein elevated in the blood-stream of patients who are either actively allergic or who have a tendency in this direction. When a high IgE level is present, it is a strong indication that the patient is allergy prone. (See page 8 for further discussion of the IgE level.)

Skin tests   Direct skin tests using the prick/puncture technique (see pages 26–28) are the best screening method we have today for evaluating a patient suspected of having a food allergy. Despite this statement I have not been impressed with any type of direct testing procedure when it comes to the question of food allergy. There are many problems associated with skin testing for food. Let me illustrate just one type of problem the allergist has to cope with: false-positive and false-negative food test results. Here are two examples: Tony, aged four, was suspected of developing hives whenever he ate food containing tomatoes. Since pizza was his favorite food it became very important to find out if he really was allergic. The prick test for tomato was negative. On his next visit, Tony was only too happy to devour a tomato, and within thirty minutes the hives appeared. This is an illustration of a false-negative test result.

On the other hand, Cindy, a nine-year-old, had been denied the pleasure of eating chocolate for many weeks. Her mother suspected that Cindy's stomach pains developed whenever she drank Coca-Cola or ate a chocolate candy bar. Her test was positive. When she was challenged with increasing amounts of cola drinks and chocolate over several days there was absolutely no discomfort. So here we have a false-positive test result.

Unfortunately, these situations occur all too frequently in the evaluation of patients suspected of having a food allergy. While these procedures may be of assistance for a small number of patients, the personal history remains the single most effective method of diagnosis.

RAST test   This is an in vitro laboratory test that has been used quite often in the evaluation of patients suspected of having food allergy. I believe that often this test is ordered very unselectively by some physicians. While an occasional patient will be an appropriate candidate for this test, most of the time I have found that the results contradicted the history. This serves to confuse rather than clarify the picture.

Management of Food Allergies

In my opinion, and in the opinion of many allergists today, the best method for both diagnosing and treating reactions to food is by dietary manipulation. What does this term mean? More or less what it implies is the addition and removal of both natural and artifiical substances from the diet, both for the purpose of diagnosing and treating symptoms caused by a suspected food or foods. Here are some of the dietary manipulation techniques I have found most effective.

Keeping a food diary Any parent whose child is suspected of having a food allergy should make use of a basic food diary. This is done by keeping a detailed list of *all* the foods and beverages—even medications and substances such as toothpaste and mouthwash—taken by the patient in the course of a day. Preferably recorded in a notebook that is kept handy day and night, the diary serves as an ongoing record of everything that has passed the child's lips at a friend's house, for lunch, dinner, snacks, at school, in front of the TV, on a hike, before bed, at the movies, whatever.

How many days or weeks should the diary be kept? It depends on the frequency of the complaints. If your child has suspected food-related symptoms every day, then a diary which covers a seven- to ten-day period will be adequate. If the problem occurs once every five to seven days, then at least a month must be spent in compiling the record.

At the end of the designated time, you and your doctor will then examine the diary to see if any identifiable patterns are present. If it is impossible to draw conclusions, there is then no reason to continue with the diary. If, on the other hand, there is a suggestion that a specific food might be causing the symptoms, then an elimination diet is the next step. An explanation of that procedure follows.

This diary approach is, of course, entirely dependent on the thoroughness of the parents' record keeping, the frequency with which the child's symptoms occur, and the physician's ability to discern a pattern in the compiled data. Table 10 shows how a sample page of a food diary might appear.

Diet restriction Certain foods are more likely than others to provoke allergic reactions in children. Highest on the list are milk, chocolate (including cola drinks), corn, citrus fruits, eggs, wheat, nuts, fish with scales, and shellfish. If you suspect that these or some other foods in particular are causing the problem, and if the symptoms occur frequently, or better yet, if they are present every day, you can try for a limited time to be your own doctor. While this evaluation must be done at home, it is best practiced under a physician's guidance.

Start by removing the food in question and any substances which contain this food from your child's diet for a period of seven to fourteen days. During this time see if the suspicious symptom has disappeared. Within a week or two you should be able to tell whether the suspected food is at fault, simply because its absence from the menu will, hopefully, coincide with the absence of the symptoms.

Next, reintroduce the food, beginning with very small portions (that is to say, half an ounce of milk, a sixth of an egg yolk) and increase the amount every day until you are giving a regular portion. If the symptoms return, the diagnostic battle is three-quarters won. To win it entirely, repeat the same process once more, making sure not to change any of the variables. If the results can be duplicated *twice,* you may be certain you have discovered the culprit. If, on the other hand, the removal of the tested food has no effect on

Table 10.   Sample Diary Entry

Date	Time Food Was Eaten	Type of Food	Reactions, if any
2/15			
	7:00 A.M.	Brushed teeth with Colgate	None
	7:15	Wheaties with milk and apple slices	None None
		Orange juice	None
	10:30	Milk and cookies	Slight stomachache
	12:30 P.M.	Spaghetti and meat sauce	None
		White bread and butter	None
		Glass of milk	None
	4:45	Chocolate candy bar	None
	6:30	Roast beef	None
		Gravy	None
		Peas	None
		French fried potatoes	None
		Glass of chocolate milk	None
	7:45	Cookies and Ovaltine	None
	8:00	Brushed teeth with Colgate	None

the symptoms one way or the other, acquit this substance and go on to another. This technique is called an *elimination diet.* If symptoms occur infrequently, it may not be feasible to use this technique for diagnosis.

General comments   Foods that cause hives and those that may cause "allergic reactions" are not necessarily synonymous. A child may develop symptoms of sneezing, runny nose, cough, wheeze, nausea or vomiting as a consequence of an allergic reaction to food. They may never exhibit any skin symptoms such as atopic dermatitis (an eczematous eruption), itching or the appearance of hives.

There is nothing wrong with a short-term do-it-yourself diet manipulation. The removal of a food or food group (i.e., dairy or citrus) from the diet for seven to fourteen days will not cause any significant nutritional disturbance. The only time there is any danger is when the initial reaction suspected of being triggered by a food was anaphylactic in nature. I don't believe that in this situation that any parent should ever be his or her own doctor!

Food challenge test   The only way to be completely certain that a particular food is causing a specific symptom is to eat that food and observe the results. The most controlled method we have for doing this is the double-blind food challenge test. Here neither the doctor nor the patient knows whether the substance about to be eaten is the suspected food or a placebo. If, for example, it is suspected that Elisabeth is getting hives from peanuts and if her symptoms have continued for several years, it is conceivable that if she just *thinks* that she is going to eat peanuts an attack will occur. If no one, neither patient nor doctor, knows whether the substance about to be eaten contains peanuts or a tolerated food, the results will be uninfluenced either by suggestion or expectation.

As a rule, challenge tests are done in hospitals or in a physician's office where emergency measures are available in case reactions turn out to be unexpectedly severe. The test food is freeze-dried to disguise its taste. It is fed to the child in an opaque capsule and the child is observed for the presence or absence of symptoms. Children too young to swallow capsules are given small amounts of the suspected substance hidden in tolerated foods.

Once challenge or elimination techniques have determined that a food allergy actually exists, treatment consists of avoiding the offending substance and its entire family of related foods. For example, if a child is allergic to milk she must also avoid butter, cream, yogurt, cheese, ice cream and milk solids in other foods. Does this mean that Susie can never eat peanut butter again, or eggs? In general, no. For most children food allergies are temporary, and except in the rare situation in which an anaphylactic reaction occurred, the cautious reintroduction of an eliminated food may begin within six to twelve months after its removal. Before taking such a step, of course, a discussion with your child's physician is in order. In general, the earlier in life the problem is detected, the greater the chances are that the specific sensitivity will disappear.

Other Possible Treatments for Food Allergies

Other forms of treatment for food problems are considerably less effective than diet regulation. Cromolyn sodium, a drug commonly prescribed for asthma and rhinitis (see the chapters on asthma and rhinitis), has been given by mouth in an attempt to treat food allergies. The amounts that must be used, however, are large and the results have not been impressive. At present cromolyn sodium has *not* been approved by the FDA for the treatment of food allergies.

Research, of course, continues on other drugs which may someday prove helpful, but to date none are ready for clinical trials. Immunotherapy and oral desensitization have from time to time been prescribed for this problem, but from my experience and the experience of most other allergists, they are not recommended for routine clinical use.

Food Additives and Allergy

Chemical substances that color, preserve, and stabilize are being added to our foods in ever-increasing numbers. While these agents are supposed to improve the condition and prolong the freshness of our food supply, they have also been responsible for causing a large number of harmful side effects. Some of these reactions can be classified as idiosyncratic or unusual reactions, and others are truly allergic in nature.

One of the major offenders in this group is a dye called tartrazine, also known as FD&C Yellow No. 5. It is found in orange, purple and green food products as well as in drugs that are colored yellow. Phenolphthalein, a related coloring derived from coal tar and used to make candy pink, can also produce adverse effects in sensitized children including headache and breathing difficulties.

Monosodium glutamate (MSG), which is used both as a flavoring agent and a meat tenderizer, is responsible for the condition known as the Chinese Restaurant Syndrome. Typical symptoms include headache, facial flushing, and chest pain.

Sodium benzoate, a preservative, has been reported to cause severe asthma symptoms in adults. It has rarely been responsible for causing problems for children.

Sensitivity to sulfites is becoming a significant problem for both pediatric and adult asthma patients. Since the late 1970's more and more fresh, frozen, and processed foods have been preserved with a variety of sulfiting agents. These include potassium bisulfite, sodium bisulfite, sodium metabisulfite, and sulfur dioxide.

With the trend toward eating natural or healthy foods more of us are heading toward the salad bars found in many restaurants. Unfortunately the sulfiting chemicals are used to preserve the freshness of many of the vegetables at the salad bar.

The most significant reactions caused by sulfite sensitivity are severe asthma and anaphylactic shock. For a list of foods and drugs treated with sulfites, check page 263 in the Appendix.

Clearly, while additives are not a major cause of allergic difficulties in children, their potential to cause adverse reactions has been well documented. The problem might not be so worrisome if food and drug manufacturers made a point of listing all additives on the labels of their products. Federal laws, unfortunately, are somewhat lax on this point, and many potentially allergy causing compounds go unannounced and hence unperceived by consumers. The only answer to this frustrating and possibly dangerous situation is for you, the consumer, to become as knowledgeable as possible regarding the specific contents of the foods and drugs used by you and your family. (For help in this effort a list of potentially allergenic additives and the foods/drugs in which they appear is provided in the Appendix.)

The Feingold Hypothesis

A discussion of the ill effects of chemical allergens would not be complete without a word regarding the famous Feingold hypothesis. In 1975, Dr. Benjamin Feingold wrote a book proclaiming that artificial dyes, colorings and food preservatives can often be the unsuspected cause of hyperactivity in children. If a child is placed on a diet free of these potentially harmful chemical substances, Feingold maintained, these hyperactive behavior patterns will soon disappear.

Extensive publicity in the lay press and on TV quickly followed Dr. Feingold's book, and for a while the Feingold diet was extremely popular, even though the program it called for required a considerable investment of time, effort and expense. The only problem with this highly attractive hypothesis was that it simply did not hold up—when rigidly controlled scientific evaluations of Dr. Feingold's theories were carried out in independent medical centers throughout the country.

What is the current thinking about Dr. Feingold's hypothesis? Most allergists would agree that only a very small percent of hyperactive children might benefit from a rigidly maintained diet free of all artificial coloring, dyes and other additives. However, the time, effort and expense involved in attempting to continue such a program over a long period (possibly years) does not make this approach a reasonable option for most families. The success rate for this diet is somewhere between 5 and 10 percent. Based on what I have said, I do not recommend this approach for my patients.

Summing Up

Despite advances in the diagnosis of suspected food allergies using such procedures as RAST testing and double-blind food challenges, clinical allergy still has a distance to go before this complicated and frustrating problem can be entirely solved. However, new diagnostic techniques are being constantly evaluated that will hopefully provide us with the necessary tools to accurately diagnose and successfully treat this problem. Meanwhile, with an approach on the part of the parents that is based on common sense and that is carried out in a logical step-by-step fashion, the great majority of children can now be helped, some to the extent that they can be kept largely symptom free.

Questions and Answers about Food Allergies

At what age may parents begin to see symptoms of food allergies in their child?

Once a child has been exposed to a food and has become sensitized to it, allergic symptoms can begin at any time. This means that foods eaten by the mother during pregnancy could conceivably sensitize the child. I have seen children display allergic reactions to their formula within the first few days of life.

Is it possible to eat a certain food for a long period of time and then suddenly become allergic to it?

Yes, a child can become allergic to a food today that she tolerated yesterday. It's a question really of how long it takes to become sensitized. For some children this process occurs after a short exposure; for others it may require years.

Are recipes available for children with food allergies? Where can this information be found?

Check the Appendix for addresses of companies which supply this information.

A child who has a severe allergic reaction to a specific food inadvertently eats this food. What should be done?

Make him throw up immediately so that all the offending food is removed from his intestinal tract. Then give him an antihistamine. Watch the child carefully for the development of symptoms. If intestinal, skin or respiratory discomfort is noted, take him to the nearest physician or emergency room for observation and possible treatment.

What relationship, if any, exists between migraine headaches and food allergies?

There does seem to be a small but definite segment of young migraine patients who suffer from food sensitivity.

Does cooked food tend to cause fewer allergic problems than raw food?

As a general rule, cooked food is less likely to trigger an allergic response than the same food uncooked. This is especially true of fruits and vegetables.

Can touching or smelling a food trigger an allergic reaction in a sensitized child?

Yes, it is possible for a young person who is highly allergic to develop symptoms merely by contact or inhalation. I once treated a three-year-old girl who was so egg-sensitive she would break out with generalized hives whenever she touched an egg, even if the egg was still in its shell. I also know of a four-year-old boy who developed severe asthmatic symptoms the moment he entered a house or restaurant where the odor of cooked fish was in the air. Such sensitivities are rare.

Are food allergies seasonal?

The only way in which the time of year might play a role is if a child has a seasonal allergy problem such as rose or hay fever. Then, when the child experiences symptoms of the seasonal allergy, the eating of a food ordinarily tolerated during a period of acute allergic symptoms may prove just the straw to break the camel's back, causing the child to react allergically to the food as well. It might also be pointed out that fruits and vegetables are by their nature seasonal. While it appears to Johnny's parents that Johnny suffers from allergies only in the late summer, this problem is actually caused (for the sake of argument) by the fact that fresh peaches, the real source of the problem, are available only at that time of year.

Can a person be allergic to common seasonings such as salt and pepper?

Pepper, along with the array of spices commonly used in our daily diet, can occasionally cause allergic problems. So can the chemical flavoring MSG (monosodium glutamate), which many cooks use to tenderize meat and enhance the flavor of vegetables. As far as I know—though anything is possible in this field—salt by itself has never been responsible for any such difficulties.

Are all foods capable of causing allergies?

While there are some foods which are quite unlikely to provoke allergic reactions such as veal and rice, there is no single substance which is totally safe. The fact is that at some time someone somewhere will develop a reaction to even the most "nonallergic" food.

Do labels on a food product list all of the ingredients found in that item?

Unfortunately, no. There are many substances, primarily chemical additives of one sort of another, which are not listed on package labels. Hopefully, legislation will soon be passed to correct this situation.

My six-month-old cannot tolerate either cow's milk or soy formula. What other choices are there?

There are a variety of specialized formulas on the market. One, MBF (meat-based formula), made by Gerber, is derived from meat. Two others, Nutramigen (Mead Johnson) and Vivonex (Norwich Eaton), contain primary essential amino acids. All of these require special preparation instructions and must be recommended by your physician.

Does a nursing mother need to watch the foods she is eating?

Definitely. Any food a mother eats will soon appear in her breast milk, even if only in small amounts. Children who are sensitized to a specific food can develop allergic symptoms this way. Nursing mothers should *always* be aware and careful of the foods they eat.

Adverse Drug Reactions

While accurate figures are difficult to obtain, it has been estimated that as many as 30 percent of hospitalized patients experience some type of adverse reaction to the drugs that they receive. Even if these figures are a bit high, the possibility of developing a drug reaction must be considered whenever a prescription is written.

What, it might then be asked, does the expression "adverse drug reaction" actually mean? Specifically, it *is a response to a drug that involves unexpected, unwanted, unpleasant symptoms.* Though many people tend to think of adverse drug reactions as being allergic, the truth is that they can stem from a variety of causes of which allergic response is just one. A comprehensive list of causes includes:

allergic reaction
intolerance
idiosyncratic reactions
overdose
side effects
drug interactions
psychogenic responses

The following imaginary conversation between a doctor and a parent is a very common occurrence.

MRS. JOHNSON: Doctor Smith, Sally has been taking penicillin now for five days—like you told her—and she's developed a bad rash.

DR. SMITH: Where's the rash located? What color is it?

MRS. JOHNSON: It's red, and it's all over her arms and legs.

DR. SMITH: Sounds like an allergy. Stop the medication right away. Sally should keep away from penicillin entirely from now on. It could be serious! I'll prescribe a different antibiotic.

In the future, penicillin may again be indicated for Sally. But when another physician attempts to prescribe it, Sally's mother will no doubt protest, regaling the doctor with horror stories of how poor Sally broke out so badly with that "allergic rash" last time she took penicillin, and how her former doctor warned that penicillin could be dangerous.

In my experience, Sally's rash and a large number of other suspected drug reactions can and often do stem from nonallergic causes. The entire subject of allergic reactions to drugs is extremely frustrating because medical technology has not yet developed accurate tests to prove whether a person is or isn't truly allergic to a specific drug. There is, however, one significant exception to this statement, and that is our ability to diagnose penicillin allergy. The point to be made here is that a diagnosis of drug allergy should not be automatically made simply from a description given over the phone. Only after a complete workup is done should a doctor diagnose a specific drug allergy.

Since we are currently not able to accurately test for possible allergy to most drugs, this diagnosis should be made after consideration has been given to *all* clinical possibilities. For example, 5 to 15 percent of patients who take a form of penicillin called Ampicillin will develop a generalized rash that is *not* an allergic reaction. If possible, the physician should examine all patients suspected of having drug reactions while physical evidence of the suspected reaction is still present. Using this information, along with the history and results of the physical examination, a doctor may be able to diagnose the cause of the reaction *without* misleading the parents concerning a nonexistent allergy.

The Many Causes of Drug Reactions

Since the difference between allergic and nonallergic drug reactions is so important for parents to understand, let's examine in detail the different types of reactions.

Allergic drug reactions   Before a drug allergy manifests itself—a reaction to penicillin, let us say—a child must first produce specific anti-IgE antibodies against that drug—i.e., *anti-penicillin IgE antibodies.* These special proteins will be found on the tissue mast cells and the basophils circulating in the bloodstream of a child who has broken out with generalized hives after taking penicillin. These antibodies can only be produced when a child has been exposed and sensitized to the specific drug. (For a complete discussion of IgE and the sensitization process, see page 8.)

Having read this statement, you may protest that your child had an allergic reactions the very first time she ever took a particular medicine. It might seem that this was the cause, but your child could have been exposed to the particular drug in question without anyone ever realizing it. For example, when a nursing mother is taking a particular medication, minute amounts of the drug are passed from her breast milk to the child. Antibiotics are occasionally put into animal feed to prevent disease. Small amounts of these substances can then pass into our food chain and hence into the diet of the child. These are only two—among many—possible sources of hidden exposure.

True allergic reactions to drugs occur in only a small percentage of the general population. There appears to be no relationship between a child's allergic reactions to things such as dust and pollen and the tendency to develop drug allergies. Even if six-year-old Nathan suffers from serious hay fever or eczema, he is, statistically speaking, no more likely to develop drug reactions than ten-year-old Brynn Elisabeth, who has never been allergic to anything in her life.

Six-year-old Ruth was given penicillin three times in her infancy and experienced no problems. The fourth time she developed serious allergic symptoms and had to be rushed to the hospital. In other words, a child who is potentially sensitive to a particular drug may have taken a drug on several previous occasions without experiencing any allergic response. The time it takes to become sensitized to a specific medication varies greatly from child to child.

Once your child is sensitized, allergic drug reactions generally occur within twenty-four hours after the drug has been taken, though delayed reactions are not unusual. As a rule, the more severe an allergic drug reaction is, the more rapid the onset of symptoms will be. An anaphylactic reaction, the most severe form of generalized allergic response, almost always begins within the first thirty to sixty minutes after the medicine enters the body. Allergic skin rashes, on the other hand, may sometimes develop as late as six or seven days after the child has taken the drug.

Once a child is sensitized to a particular drug, even minute amounts of it can trigger a reaction.

A child who develops allergic symptoms to one drug is likely to react in a similar way to other drugs derived from the same chemical family. This is particularly true of penicillin-related preparations.

Symptoms of allergic drug reactions usually subside within four to six days after the drug has been discontinued. On infrequent occasions a drug reaction may continue for many weeks. In extremely rare cases it may last for months.

Tests for penicillin and insulin sensitivity are after-the-fact procedures—there are no reliable *prospective* testing methods presently available—and screening procedures for drug allergy in general are presently quite limited.

The ultimate test is to readminister the drug to the child and note its effects. This type of challenge test is of course potentially *quite dangerous;* if it is to be considered at all, it must be done in a medical facility where treatment for a severe reaction can be quickly rendered. In most instances it is unnecessary to perform this risky procedure. Later in this chapter I will discuss specific desensitization techniques that offer another alternative.

The route by which a drug enters the body, by mouth, injection or topically through the skin, is a critical factor in determining whether that drug will cause allergic sensitization. Topical application is the route most likely to produce sensitization. Oral administration, perhaps surprisingly, is the least likely. Topical preparations containing antibiotics and antihistamines are especially prone to cause problems, and presently a number of over-the-counter preparations include *both* classes of drugs. Do not use them indiscriminately. Speak with your doctor if you have any questions.

Intolerance   First on the list of nonallergic drug reactions is a condition known as drug intolerance. Simply stated, drug intolerance refers to an unexpected increase in the *usual* activity of a drug. For example, we know that if you take double or triple the average dose of aspirin for several days, almost everyone will develop tinnitus, more commonly known as a ringing in the ears. Someone who is intolerant of aspirin would develop tinnitus after taking only one or two aspirin tablets, a normal dose. What we have is a quantitative increase in the pharmacologic action of the drug. There is no way to predict whether or not this type of reaction will occur.

Generally speaking, there is no way to control drug intolerance. Some children just can't tolerate any amount of a certain drug. A substitute preparation will have to be prescribed.

Idiosyncratic drug response   If Jenny takes an aspirin to relieve her headache and develops a blood condition called hemolytic anemia, she has had an idiosyncratic reaction: an unexpected effect that is different from the normal action of the drug. Such responses occur only in a susceptible population—the likelihood of many people developing them is small—and most symptoms are based on an unusual metabolic response rather than an immune one. Medications that produce idiosyncratic responses should *never* be given to susceptible patients, even in the smallest doses.

Drug overdose   Allergic drug reactions, drug intolerance and drug idiosyncrasy occur only among people who have a biological tendency to develop such conditions. The symptoms of drug overdose require no such predisposing susceptibility: it can happen to anyone, on purpose or by accident. The symptoms are toxic, not allergic, and can range from uncomfortable to fatal. The problem is avoided by monitoring drug intake, by careful medicating procedures, and by keeping all medicine away from very young children. Always read medication instructions carefully and ask your physician about the medicines prescribed for your child.

Side effects of drugs   We are all familiar with the phenomenon of side effects, those unwanted extra symptoms which accompany the expected pharmacologic activity of a drug. A frequent example is the headache, jittery feeling, tremor and rapid heartbeat that follow an injection of epinephrine (Adrenalin) for acute asthma. Side effects are the most common form of adverse drug reactions, more frequent by far than either drug intolerance or allergy. Many people come into my office and tell me that they are allergic to a certain antibiotic. "Why do you think you're allergic to it?" I ask. "Because when I take it I get an upset stomach," they reply. "My doctor said I'm allergic."

Nine times out of ten this problem is merely an annoying side effect and has nothing to do with an allergic reaction. Nor is such a reaction always unwanted or negative. Antihistamines produce drowsiness, making them unsuitable for children who must remain alert in school. At bedtime, the antihistamine's soporific effect can be a blessing, helping children to relax as it relieves their sneezing and itching. Many sedative drugs on the market today actually contain an antihistamine as a primary ingredient.

Side effects can be coped with in several ways, changing the dosage and altering the frequency of administration being the two most common. In some situations nothing can be done to help, and then the medication must simply be changed.

Interactions between drugs When a child takes more than one medication at a time, the possibility always exists that the two will not mix and might produce unexpected and unwanted reactions. It is advisable to check with your child's doctor or local pharmacist regarding the possibility of a reaction when more than one drug is being prescribed. To accommodate this problem many pharmacists, especially those in the larger pharmacies or chain drugstores, use computers to check whether a specific combination of drugs is likely to cause potential problems for the patient. This type of service will become more comprehensive as the technology becomes more readily available.

Coincidental response As part of their natural course many viral illnesses produce a rash. If a child happens to be taking any medication at the same time, especially an antibiotic, the drug may be accused of causing the rash. In reality, it is a natural response to the virus itself and has nothing to do with the medicine. The problem is that there is no easy way to perform a test and then declare, "Yes, Johnny's problem is the medication," or, "No, the medication had nothing to do with Johnny's rash; the virus caused it." All a parent can do in this situation is to be informed that the possibility exists of mistaking one causative factor for another, and to report all suspicious symptoms to the doctor.

Psychogenic reactions I have seen children become dizzy or even pass out after receiving an injection. Almost always this reaction is psychologically triggered, based either on fear of pain or terror of the needle. Rarely if ever is it a specific response to the injected material.

Despite the fact that these reactions are psychological rather than physiological, I have heard parents claim that their child experienced a severe allergic reaction while at the doctor's office—even after the matter had been thoroughly explained, and seemingly understood. As for the physician, it is important for him to find out if the child has ever had any previous reactions to injections; if a child is particularly frightened by needles, he should be approached with care. The doctor should explain in clear, simple language what he is going to do and the child should be told what type of examination will be done before the office visit. I have found it particularly helpful to illustrate this explanation by giving the first injection (a placebo, of course) to one of the parents. Quite often this example will calm and reassure the child that nothing terrible is going to happen. The time spent in this careful approach will yield dividends in terms of a more cooperative patient and, in general, a better doctor-patient relationship.

Identifying Allergic Drug Reactions

What type of reaction might one expect if the response is in fact allergic? There are four varieties.

Anaphylactic response   This frightening reaction is rapid in onset and simultaneously involves many parts of the body including the skin, lungs, and cardiovascular system. Before it can take place, as with all allergic reactions, previous exposure and sensitization to the offending drug must have occurred. Common symptoms include:

hives
generalized itchy rash
angioedema: swelling of the face involving the lips, tongue, and eyes
nasal discharge, sneezing
shortness of breath, wheezing
drop in blood pressure and rapid heartbeat

The reaction can begin immediately following injection of medication, but more commonly the symptoms occur within thirty to sixty minutes after the drug enters the body.

Cytotoxic response   This reaction requires the presence of another class of antibodies, called IgG, in the bloodstream. These antibodies attach to the surface of red blood cells and ultimately lead to their destruction (cytotoxic means "cell destroying"). When large numbers of red blood cells are destroyed, a person becomes anemic. The drugs that can trigger a cytotoxic reaction include the sulfa drugs, various antibiotics and certain anticonvulsant agents. This is not a frequent occurrence.

Immune complex–mediated drug reaction   Immune complex reactions occur when large collections of antigens and antibodies are deposited in the skin, blood vessels, kidneys and central nervous system as a result of an allergic response to a drug. The classic example of this phenomenon is a condition called serum sickness, which has the following symptoms:

hives
an itchy, slightly raised rash
swollen, painful joints
tender lymph nodes
fever

This type of allergic response was much more common when vaccines were prepared from horse serum. Today animal serums are rarely used in the manufacture of biologic vaccines, and the most common cause of immune complex reactions is penicillin. Serum sickness usually takes from seven to fourteen days to develop. The average duration of symptoms is approximately seven days, but the clinical picture can last for several weeks. Chances for complete recovery are excellent.

Delayed allergic response   Contact dermatitis is the most common symptom of a delayed allergic drug reaction. Probably the best example of this type of reaction is the rash associated with poison ivy. Many drugs applied topically are also responsible for causing contact dermatitis. Symptoms can take from three to seven days to develop.

Another variation on this theme is a response to light called a photosensitivity reaction. In some individuals the combination of certain chemical substances (called photoallergens) and exposure to ultraviolet light, from either the sun or an artificial source, causes a photoallergic or a phototoxic rash. The drugs most commonly involved in this reaction include the sulfonamides, griseofulvin (an antifungal drug) and chlorothiazide (a diuretic). Common photoallergens are chemicals found in hair tonics, sunscreens, antiseptic soaps, certain lipstick dyes, and topical antibiotics. The most important method of treating a photosensitivity reaction is avoiding the trouble-causing chemicals.

Diagnosing Drug Allergies

In reviewing the different responses that might result from a drug reaction, it becomes clear that the common allergic symptoms—sneezing, wheezing, and hives—make up only a part of the possible spectrum of reactions. After this review of a list of these potential responses, let's find out how the allergist attempts to evaluate them.

Preparing for the Medical History

The starting point is always a detailed medical history. Everything the family and the child can remember concerning the reaction should be reviewed during the first visit with the doctor. Because of the limited number of testing procedures available for evaluating drug allergies, this history is especially critical. Things you may wish to tell the doctor include:

What drug or drugs has the child taken, and in what dose?

What previous exposure, if any, has the child had to the suspected drug or a related class of drugs?

How long after the medicine was given did the symptoms become noticeable?

Describe the symptoms.

How long do the symptoms last?

What treatment, if any, was given? What was the response to treatment?

When the suspected medication was discontinued, what changes, if any, were noted in the child's symptoms? How long did it take for the symptoms to clear up?

Test Procedures

Once the history and physical examination have been completed, the doctor will then have to decide if he can use the medical laboratory to help him make the diagnosis. The unfortunate situation that currently exists is the lack of available specific testing procedures to evaluate most suspected allergic drug reactions. The problem facing research scientists who are trying to develop these testing procedures is that when a drug enters the body many breakdown products are formed. Any one or combination of these biologically active compounds may then be responsible for the suspected allergic reaction. But which ones? That's the question. Putting the pieces of the puzzle into place is a formidable process and so far scientists have been able to accomplish this task for only a small number of medicines. One of the drugs for which a test has been developed is penicillin.

The following list includes those tests which have proven most effective in determining drug sensitivity.

Direct skin tests   Direct, in vivo procedures are available for a very limited number of drugs. These include tests for egg-containing vaccines, penicillin, insulin, and tetanus toxoid. A positive response develops within twenty minutes and consists of a raised, itchy wheal at the site of the prick or puncture. (For specific details on direct skin testing, see page 26.)

Patch tests   Patch tests are used to determine if a particular drug is causing contact dermatitis. For this test a sample of the drug (antigen) is placed directly on the patient's back or forearm and the test site is covered with an adhesive patch. It is then examined after forty-eight hours. The presence of an irritation with redness and small blisters at the test site is a positive response. This type of test does *not* provide information for symptoms caused by oral medications. (For further information on patch testing see page 28.)

In vitro or laboratory tests   The only in vitro test (i.e., test done in the laboratory) now available for drug sensitivity is the radioallergosorbert test (RAST).

The RAST test (see page 25) is presently used for the detection of penicillin allergy; no other drugs can be evaluated with this procedure. Since this test is not performed directly on the patient, it does have the obvious advantage of being risk free.

Challenge test   In this test a drug suspected of causing an allergic reaction is administered directly to the patient. If a reaction follows, it proves without question that the child is allergic to the tested drug. Such an approach can of course be highly dangerous and should be attempted only under strict medical supervision. Challenge testing for drugs, on the whole, is rarely indicated.

Identifying Allergic Reactions to Specific Drugs

One basic fact must be stated at the beginning of this section. Based solely on a child's physical signs and symptoms there is no way that either you as the parent or I as the physician can identify the specific cause of an adverse drug reaction. A doctor cannot examine a youngster and then tell the parent which drug is responsible for the symptoms. While certain types of reactions may be more frequently associated with one drug or another, there is no truly consistent pattern when it comes to the confusing world of drug reactions.

Penicillin

In the four decades since penicillin was discovered, it has been one of the safest drugs available to doctors today. Billions of doses have been prescribed through the years with proportionately few serious side effects. And yet, safe as it is, penicillin is so widely prescribed that it is responsible for the majority of drug-induced anaphylactic deaths in this country, a figure estimated to run somewhere between three hundred and seven hundred fatalities a year.

What symptoms can be caused by an allergic reaction to penicillin? The response may be localized or generalized, a relatively minor inconvenience or a potential catastrophe! The degree of response can range from an itchy contact dermatitis rash to the life-threatening symptoms of anaphylactic shock. (For a discussion of anaphylactic shock, see the chapter on allergic emergencies, page 243).

At times penicillin reactions will be delayed, occurring from six to eight days after treatment has begun, usually in the form of hives or serum sickness with the following symptoms: fever, rash, swollen lymph nodes, joint swelling, pain and angioedema. Still another reaction occasionally associated with penicillin is hemolytic anemia, which results from the destruction of red blood cells. Fortunately, this condition is very uncommon, and is especially rare in childhood.

By far the most frequent reaction to penicillin is a measles-like rash consisting of small, slightly raised areas that are found mainly on the arms, legs and trunk. The skin lesions may range in color from a pale pink to purple. The rash generally clears without specific treatment within fourteen to twenty-one days. The exact cause of this reaction is unknown. It may be toxic and nonallergic in nature. Note, too, that certain penicillin derivatives such as Ampicillin will cause a maculopapular rash in 5 to 15 percent of people. This response is a side effect of the drug and not a true allergic reaction. If your child develops a rash while taking Ampicillin, then it will be necessary to have specific penicillin allergy testing done. This is the only way to determine whether the rash was a true allergic reaction or merely an unwanted, confusing side effect of this drug.

When penicillin enters the body, it is metabolized into a number of breakdown products, the two main components being the major and the minor determinants. An allergic reaction to either one or both of these breakdown products is responsible for the clinical symptoms of penicillin sensitivity. Testing should always be done for both major and minor determinants. A positive response to the minor determinant mixture tells the doctor that your child is at risk of developing an anaphylactic reaction from penicillin. A positive reaction to the major determinant indicates that a rapid onset of generalized hives is likely to occur.

The test procedure consists of a series of skin tests using both prick and intradermal techniques. Both the major determinant and the minor determinant mixture are tested first with the prick technique, and if that is negative, intradermal testing is performed. A positive reaction consists of a red, raised, itchy area at the test site which develops within twenty minutes.

What happens if your child tests positively for penicillin allergy but nevertheless must take this drug to cure a life-threatening infection? In such a situation it is possible to desensitize the patient by employing either an oral or intravenous technique. The patient is started on minute amounts of the drug and the dosage is slowly increased over a period of eight to twelve hours until it reaches a therapeutic dose. This procedure provides immunity only on a temporary basis by overwhelming the body's capacity to react allergically only while the child is receiving the drug. When the penicillin is stopped, the sensitivity will return within two or three days. This means that if penicillin must be given again, the complete desensitization process must be repeated. Desensitization programs must be carried out under direct medical supervision preferably in a hospital setting where emergency treatment is available.

There are a few last important points concerning penicillin sensitivity.

Skin testing for penicillin should be done only for patients who are suspected of having had a previous reaction to this drug or a related antibiotic.

Penicillin allergy is not hereditary. The fact that Aunt Rita and cousin Tommy are allergic to Ampicillin does not mean that your child is at an increased risk.

Studies have shown that only 10 to 20 percent of people who are suspected of having penicillin allergy show a positive response when tested for it. Many people who think they are allergic to penicillin actually tolerate it quite well.

Orally administered penicillin is less prone to cause an allergic reaction than the same drug given intravenously or by injection.

If a skin test is positive, it means there is a very good chance that an allergic reaction will develop if penicillin is taken. If the test is *negative,* this is by no means a guarantee that the patient cannot at some future time become sensitive to this drug.

Aspirin (Acetyl Salicylic Acid)

In the United States, approximately 30 million pounds of aspirin are consumed every year; that's a lot of little white pills! Because of its widespread use it ranks second only to penicillin as a cause of adverse drug reactions. A conservative estimate would be that one million people are "allergic" to aspirin. A more accurate term to describe the actual mechanism responsible for the symptoms caused by aspirin would be "idiosyncrasy." The reaction is a qualitatively abnormal response to the drug, and no definite allergic response patterns have been found.

What should make you suspect that Johnny has a problem with aspirin? By far the most common symptom caused by a reaction to aspirin is the appearance of hives and/or angioedema. Children over the age of ten seem to have these symptoms much more frequently than their younger brothers and sisters.

There is a condition called the "aspirin triad" consisting of severe bronchial asthma, sinusitis, and nasal polyps; it is found in people with a sensitivity to aspirin. Fortunately, this syndrome is almost exclusively a problem for adults. Although a few cases have been reported in children as young as ten, they are extremely rare.

However, a word of caution. If your child has symptoms of chronic rhinitis and is diagnosed as having nasal polyps, stop using aspirin! Another group of drugs to avoid are those known as nonsteroidal anti-inflammatory drugs (NSAID), which cross-react with aspirin. The NSAID are commonly used to treat headaches, muscular pains and arthritis symptoms. The most common members of this ever-growing group are:

Alcolofenac (Mervan)
Azapropazone (Rheumox)
Diclofenac (Voltarol)
Diflunisal (Dolobid)
Fenclofenac (Flenac)
Fenoprofen (Nalfon)
Feprazone (Methrazone)
Ibuprofen (Motrin)

Indomethacin (Indocin)
Mefenamic acid (Ponstel)
Naproxen (Naprosyn)
Oxyphenbutazone (Oxalid, Tandearil)
Sulindac (Clinoril)
Tolmetin (Tolectin, Rufen)
Zomepirac (Zomax)

As substitutes for the aspirin-sensitive person the following drugs may be used:

Acetaminophen (Tylenol, Datril)   Salicylamide (Os-Cal-Gesic)
Choline magnesium trisalicylate (Tri-   Salicylsalicylic acid (Disalcid)
    lisate)   Sodium salicylate (Pabalate)
Choline salicylate (Arthropan)
Propoxyphene hydrochloride (Dar-
    von)

Approximately 15 percent of aspirin-sensitive patients also react to a dye known as tartrazine or FD&C Yellow No. 5. (For a complete list of tartrazine-containing substances, see the Appendix.)

There are no available tests which can be done to prove that a person is sensitive to aspirin. A direct challenge test can be done, but as I have stated before, this is potentially dangerous and must be carried out only under direct medical supervision.

Finally, in instances where a child has had a reaction to aspirin but where aspirin is absolutely essential for the treatment of a specific medical problem —as in some forms of juvenile rheumatoid arthritis or in rheumatic fever— a method of desensitization is available similar to that used for penicillin (see above). Once desensitization has been carried out, however, aspirin will be tolerated only as long as it is given on a continuous basis and, as with penicillin desensitization, the allergic sensitivity will return when the drug is discontinued.

Local Anesthetics

Adverse reactions to local anesthetic agents occur most commonly in the dentist's chair, especially after a child has received an injection of a painkiller such as Xylocaine. Reactions can range from mild discomfort to a life-threatening emergency and may stem from toxic responses, psychological causes, or allergic reactions.

Allergic reactions are the least frequent of the three. Ordinarily they consist of a contact sensitivity, an itch or rash. Usually they are caused by a topical over-the-counter cream or ointment, an anti-itch preparation, for instance, or a hemorrhoid salve that contains anesthetics. Generally speaking, allergic reactions to injected local anesthetics are very unusual.

Toxic reactions are more frequent. These are due to several possible mechanisms: unknowingly injecting the anesthetic into a blood vessel, intolerance to a normally absorbed drug or possibly overdosage due to ultra-rapid absorption of the drug. Symptoms occur when the medication reaches the central nervous and cardiovascular systems.

The most common story is: Susie went to the dentist and received an injection of a painkiller; then the trouble began. Symptoms may consist of

Table 11.   Acetaminophen Drugs

Name	Form
Acetaminophen	Tablet
Acetaminophen Uniserts	Suppository
Comtrex	Tablets
Congesprin Liquid Cold Medicine	Liquid
Contac Jr. Children's Cold Medicine	Liquid
Coricidin Sinus Headache Tablets	Tablets
CoTylenol Liquid Cough Formula	Liquid
Datril	Tablets
Excedrin	Tablets
Liquiprin	Liquid
Novahistine Sinus Tablets	Tablets
Ornex Capsules	Capsule
Phenaphen	Capsule
Sine-Aid Sinus Headache Tablets	Tablets
Sinutab Tablets	Tablets
Tempra	Drops
Trind	Liquid
Tylenol Regular Strength	Tablet
Tylenol Extra Strength	Liquid
Vanquish	Caplet

slurred speech, restlessness, dizziness, nausea, vomiting, confusion progressing to convulsions, coma, a drop in blood pressure, cardiac failure and possibly death.

By far the most frequent type of reaction to a topical anesthetic agent is caused by a vasovagal response. Here just the *thought* of a dental appointment or impending surgery can precipitate dizziness, palpitations and fainting. The condition is, in short, a psychological reaction, one which in many cases can be helped best by discussing the anxiety with your doctor or dentist.

Finally, note that local anesthetics can be divided into two groups which chemically are quite different from one another. It would be quite unusual for a person to have an allergic reaction to members of both these groups. If a child has a reaction to an anesthetic from one of these groups, the doctor will normally substitute a drug from the second, usually with complete success. If there is concern that a child has had reactions to both groups of anesthetic agents, then direct skin testing can be performed; however, the results are not absolutely diagnostic.

X-Ray Contrast Media

Today many specialized X-ray studies require the intravenous injection of iodine-containing compounds called radiographic contrast media (RCM). In approximately 5 percent of patients who are tested, adverse reactions occur within three minutes following the injection of the contrast media. Although extremely unusual, it is possible to develop kidney failure within twenty-four hours of the injection.

The exact reason why these reactions develop is not clear. A true allergic mechanism has only rarely been proven and most reactions have been labeled as anaphylactoid.

The usual symptoms associated with this response are hives, a drop in blood pressure, angioedema, wheezing and shock. Other findings have included vomiting, nausea, tingling sensations of the arms and legs, and profuse sweating.

Unfortunately, there are deaths associated with these procedures; the statistics approximate the frequency to be somewhere between 1 in 10,000 to 1 in 400,000 patients receiving contrast media injections. However, the vast majority of contrast media reactions are mild and of very short duration.

Table 12. Local Anesthetics

Group A		Group B	
Generic Name	Brand Name	Generic Name	Brand Name
Procaine	Novocain	Lidocaine	Xylocaine
Benzocaine	—	Mepivacaine	Carbocaine
Tetracaine	Pontocaine	Dibucaine	Nupercaine
Chloroprocaine	Nesacaine	Phenacaine	Holocaine
Butethamine	Monocaine	Cyclomethycaine	Surtacaine
Butacaine	Butyn	Hexylcaine	Cyclaine
Larocaine	—	Cocaine	—

NOTE: In general, reactions to agents in group A will not occur if a group B drug is substituted or vice versa.

While there is certainly reason to be absolutely sure that an X-ray study is necessary before going ahead with it, the possibility of an adverse reaction occurring from the RCM is extremely small. And when a reaction to contrast media does take place, children appear to be at far less risk than adults.

At present no foolproof pretest exists to determine whether a patient will have an adverse reaction to RCM. The best that can be offered is the administration of a small trial dose of the dye immediately before the test begins. If the patient shows no adverse reactions to this sample, then a full dose can be given, *usually*—but not always—safely. Another approach especially for patients who have had a reaction in the past involves the administration of both cortisone and the antihistamine Benadryl twenty-four hours before the test is performed, though once again this procedure helps some but not all patients. Fortunately, with the advent of newer imaging techniques such as the CAT scan and Magnetic Resonance Imaging (MRI), the frequency with which contrast media studies are performed will be decreasing, and no doubt there will be a proportional drop in the number of adverse reactions as a result.

Insulin

While diabetes certainly is not infrequent among children, the majority of adverse insulin responses occur in adults. Reactions to insulin run the gamut from local skin eruptions to generalized anaphylaxis, though just how prevalent these reactions are is difficult to determine. In the medical literature, estimates of insulin sensitivity have ranged from as low as 1 percent to as high as 50 percent. Significantly, it is known that approximately one-tenth of all diabetic patients will at some time require changes in their insulin therapy; that's a pretty good indication that insulin sensitivity is not a negligible factor among the diabetic population.

Types of allergic insulin reactions include the following:

Wheal and flare   This skin response starts within two to three weeks after insulin therapy is begun. Symptoms consist of local redness (flares) and swelling (wheals) at the injection site. Ordinarily they appear fifteen minutes after the dose has been given and then disappear within two to three hours.

Late-phase response   Some diabetics develop a wheal and flare response locally, three to six hours after the insulin has been administered. The involved area becomes red and quite painful. It clears within twenty-four hours.

Delayed reaction   Delayed reactions appear eight to twelve hours after injection. They are characterized by itchy, well-outlined, painful and slightly swollen areas at the injection site. Discomfort increases hourly, reaching its peak in twenty-four hours. The condition usually takes several days to disappear entirely.

Generalized reaction   This response is infrequent but may be quite severe when it occurs. It can include hives, itching, angioedema and shock.

For patients prone to allergic insulin responses, switching from pork to beef insulin or to a more purified variety of insulin will often solve the problem. In some cases, insulin desensitization procedures are also appropriate. A diabetes specialist or an allergist can provide you with information regarding these specialized techniques.

Prevention, Treatment and Control of Allergic Drug Reactions

Avoidance

If your child has had some form of adverse reaction to a specific drug, avoidance is by far the best—and often the only—treatment. Problems arise because it is generally impossible to know in advance which drugs will trigger adverse reactions, how these reactions will affect your child and which medicines on the market contain the harmful drug. This is especially true if the drug in question happens to be a common one such as aspirin.

Still, certain steps can be taken:

Copy down the names of any medicine your child has reacted to in the past. Do not rely on the doctor to keep these records for you. Even if your doctor has such information on file, the physician may not always be available when the data is needed. Keep your own records. Carefully update them as required.

As soon as your child reaches responsible age, she should be given all pertinent information regarding drugs and/or foods containing the allergenic substance. If parents and child work together on this project, prevention can become a successful family affair.

Whenever the information is available, familiarize yourself with those drugs that interreact adversely with one another. It is important to know that an aspirin-sensitive asthmatic child should avoid foods and medicines which contain tartrazine dyes. At the same time, with the flood of new medications on the market the subject of cross-reactions among drugs is becoming so complicated that it is virtually impossible to keep track of them all. Fortunately, as mentioned above, many pharmacies are meeting this need with computers that provide information on both cross-reactive drugs and unacceptable drug combinations.

When adverse drug reactions do occur, treatment with antihistamines, adrenaline, bronchodilators and, when necessary, cortisone will almost always control symptoms.

Get into the habit of reading the labels on all medicine bottles before giving the medication to your child. If you have any questions about whether a particular offending chemical is contained in these medicines, consult with your physician and/or contact the drug company directly.

If your child is sensitive to a particular drug, it may be wise to have him wear a name tag and keep an identification card in his wallet identifying the specific allergy and/or the problematic drug. Metal wristbands or necklaces identifying the allergy are also useful. While a number of companies market these items, perhaps the best known is the Medic Alert bracelet, information on which can be obtained from your physician or from most pharmacies.

Provocative Drug Testing

If no test is available to confirm a possible drug sensitivity ana it is *absolutely necessary* to use the drug, then it may become necessary to perform a challenge test. This means that a small dose of the suspect medication is given the child who is then closely watched *in* the physician's office for several hours. Such a test is not without some risk, and the decision to perform a challenge test must be based both on the severity of the child's original reaction as well as the unavailability of a nonrelated drug that would be equally effective in treating the condition.

Desensitization

This therapeutic technique has been discussed and described throughout this chapter. Currently it is available for a limited number of drugs including aspirin, penicillin and insulin. The point to be made here again is that desensitization to a drug is *always* temporary and lasts only as long as the child continues to receive the medication. Despite this drawback, however, desensitization does represent the only really satisfactory way we have of safely administering an absolutely necessary drug to a needy allergic patient, and its enormous value should be obvious to everyone.

Questions and Answers about Drug Allergies

Is there any relationship between drug allergies and the seasons of the year?

No, seasonal patterns do not in any way affect allergic drug responses. A person who is sensitive to a specific medicine in the snows of February will react just as readily to this drug in the heat of July.

What should be done if a child who is reputedly allergic to tetanus toxoid steps on a rusty nail?

In the case of a child with a *proven* allergy to tetanus toxoid, a special tetanus antitoxin can be used. This substance is made from material prepared from human rather than horse serum. It is also possible to do a skin test for tetanus toxoid ahead of time to check for the possibility of allergy. If the test is negative, the immunization can then be performed without worry. True allergic reactions to tetanus toxoid, it should be added, are extremely rare.

Can a child die from serum sickness?

Serum sickness, a condition that develops following the administration of an animal serum (such as horse serum) or a drug (such as penicillin), rarely if ever ends in death. Still, the symptoms can sometimes be severe. They include fever, hives and painful joints which usually develop anywhere from six to ten days after the medication or animal serum has been administered. The condition usually clears within one to two weeks. Rarely, the symptoms may linger for more than a month.

Can any medicine cause an allergic reaction?

Yes. Certainly some drugs have an especially low allergic risk associated with them. Yet a doctor can never say with absolute assurance that any drug is 100 percent safe.

Can a drug reaction ever produce permanent effects?

On the whole the chances are exceedingly rare. Still, one must never say "never" when talking about medicine. For instance, there is an unlikely possibility that the blood, bone marrow and neurological system of a child may be affected by certain unusual drug reactions, with resultant organ damage and long-term lingering problems. These cases make up such a tiny percentage of the total number of drug reactions, however, that they are worth mentioning only to keep the record straight.

Is it true that once a child becomes allergic to a drug she will always be allergic to it?

If a child is truly allergic to a medication and does not simply have an idiosyncratic or toxic reaction, chances are that her sensitivity will last. A good general recommendation is to keep the child away from any drugs that have been a proven cause of allergic trouble in the past. Hopefully in the coming years we will possess an increased number of accurate testing methods for drug allergies. Until then, caution is the rule.

Are drug sensitivities inherited?

There is no evidence to indicate that they are. There may be certain situations in which a specific enzyme is genetically absent from an entire population of people, causing this group to be incapable of tolerating a specific drug. An example is the primaquine-induced hemolytic anemia found in people deficient in the enzyme glucose 6-phosphate dehydrogenase. Given normal circumstances, allergies to common drugs such as aspirin or penicillin are not inherited.

Allergic Skin Conditions

An allergist is often called upon to see children with a variety of skin rashes suspected of "being caused by an allergy." The most frequent dermatologic problem I have encountered in my practice is a form of eczema called atopic dermatitis. Other frequently seen rashes belong to the category of contact dermatitis, which has many possible causes. Probably the best example of this rash is rhus dermatitis, more commonly known as poison ivy. In this chapter I will concentrate on atopic and contact dermatitis and only touch briefly on other skin conditions.

Eczema

Susan, aged three, was carried into my office in her mother's arms. Unable to extend her arms and legs, she kept them tightly flexed close to her body. Her fingers were clenched into fists and the skin on her face was as red and rough as the skin of a sailor. Her mother smiled sadly. "Eczema," she said, "and today is one of her better days."

Adam was six years old when he first came to see me. He sat in the chair opposite mine. During the entire visit he proceeded to itch, dig and literally tear at the irritating skin eruptions covering a good part of his little body. "He's always like this," his mother informed me. "It never stops!"

Jane was only two years old when her mother brought her to my office. Jane's pediatrician had noticed a small reddish patch on her cheeks some weeks earlier. He sent her to me for a diagnosis. By the time Jane arrived, the patch had almost doubled in size. "I tried to stop her from scratching it," both parents told me, "but short of putting her into a straitjacket there was just nothing we could do!"

Three different children, three different variations on the same theme. It's called eczema. And while it is not a life-threatening menace, it can be one of the most agonizing ailments imaginable. What is it exactly?

Technically speaking, eczema is not a disease at all but a reactive response of the skin. When it is restricted to a single area of the body—usually in the form of small, well-outlined, coin-sized patches that break down easily when scratched, ooze, then finally crust over—the condition is known as nummular eczema. When the eczematous rash spreads across the body and forms larger, thickened, purplish-red lesions over sheetlike areas, as it frequently does, it becomes generalized eczema. The rash is characteristically found in the bends of the elbows, on the neck and face, behind the ears, and at the backs of the knees. The appearance of the skin itself may change considerably during the various stages of the disorder: acute, chronic and subacute.

Acute stage   Characterized by redness, swelling and, when the skin has been broken, a wet, watery look called "weeping." These open skin surfaces provide an excellent breeding ground for bacteria and the development of infection. This occurs quite frequently.

Chronic stage   In its more advanced stages, after the weeping has dried, the rash takes on a dry, dark, thickened, scaling and leathery appearance.

Subacute stage   Includes characteristics of both the acute and chronic stages.

Atopic Dermatitis

Atopic dermatitis is the most common form of childhood eczema. It strikes approximately 1 to 3 percent of all infants during their first two years of life and continues to lurk as a threat for youngsters of all ages into the teenage years. Among eczema sufferers a strong family history of allergy is quite common—eczema is most likely hereditary—and figures show that a sizable percentage of atopic dermatitis patients have other allergies. Approximately 40 to 50 percent of children with atopic dermatitis develop hay fever, and between 15 and 30 percent are asthmatic. The good news is that roughly half of atopic dermatitis sufferers will spontaneously lose their eczema before becoming adults, and a majority of the remaining percentage have an excellent chance of controlling their condition.

How to Identify Atopic Dermatitis

Although most allergists agree that atopic dermatitis is an allergic condition, it is ordinarily quite difficult to pinpoint the specific causes of the problem. Certainly for a significant number of children, foods play a role, either as a primary triggering agent or as a secondary aggravating factor. By both clinical observation and the use of such procedures as the prick skin tests (see page

26) or the RAST test (see page 25), it is occasionally possible to prove that a specific food sensitivity is responsible for the atopic dermatitis. Unfortunately, this does not happen too often. In fact, much to the chagrin and frustration of the physician, atopic dermatitis is most often brought under control entirely *without* knowledge on the doctor's part of what actually caused it.

So strong is the itch associated with atopic dermatitis in some young patients that several decades ago it was not unusual to walk into the children's ward of a hospital and see infants with severe eczema with their arms and legs loosely held in restraints, the theory being that if the patients were kept from scratching their skin, the rash would subside. Because of the potentially harmful psychological effects which could develop from this treatment, it was finally abandoned. Still, the point was well made, and should be well made here: there is no doubt that if scratching is prevented in a child suffering from atopic dermatitis, even the worst eczematous rash can often be made to disappear completely. A prominent dermatologist stated that with atopic dermatitis, "It isn't the eruption that itches but the itch that erupts." The moral is that if you control the itch, you control the rash.

Atopic dermatitis can be identified by its red lesions, dry skin and intense itching. The primary task of both parents and physicians when faced with the taxing problem of the child with atopic dermatitis is to closely monitor all symptoms and get appropriate treatment as soon as possible. I will detail below some of the specific methods by which these tasks can be accomplished.

The Stages of Atopic Dermatitis

Infantile stage—up to two years of age   Though clinical symptoms of atopic dermatitis almost never appear before the age of one month, the majority of children develop their symptoms during the first year of life. Once the rash has become apparent, certain environmental conditions can aggravate the situation immensely. Winter—with its dry, cold air, heavy, irritating clothing and reduction of direct skin exposure to sunlight—is a particularly rough time for most eczema sufferers. Symptoms also seem to intensify when a youngster has a mild cold, is teething or is going through a stressful period. Curiously, some children with atopic dermatitis actually experience a *decrease* in rash symptoms when suffering from measles or other viral illness. We are not sure why this is so.

The earliest signs of atopic dermatitis usually appear on the face, especially on the cheeks, in the form of a patchy red rash. If this mild eruption is not vigorously treated, it can spread with shocking speed. I have seen a number of cases in which a small outbreak begins innocently enough on the face and then proceeds to spread over most of the body in less than a month. This type of generalized spreading can become so severe that it makes the child who was previously an angel and a delight turn into a weeping, restless, miserable waif who finds neither an hour's relief nor a moment's peace.

Not every child, of course, develops widespread rashes. I have seen many instances where only the cheeks are involved; interestingly enough, the nose and area around the mouth almost always seem to be spared. In addition to lesions on the cheeks, eczema frequently involves the backs of the ears, producing deep cracks that ooze and bleed. Other affected areas include the neck, scalp, arms, sides of the legs and the ankles. Regardless of where the rash is located, I can't recall ever seeing a patient with atopic dermatitis who didn't have severe itching. A cardinal rule to bear in mind: if the rash does not itch, it isn't atopic dermatitis.

Childhood stage—from age two through twelve   Children with eczema between the ages of two and twelve usually have very dry skin with localized lesions that tend to form in the creases and the flexed parts of the arms, neck and legs. The skin behind the ears is another commonly involved area.

Because of the persistent itch and chronic scratching associated with eczema, the skin tends to become tough and thickened with an almost leathery consistency that is rough to the touch (skin in this condition is described as being lichenified). Children whose eczema persists into the school years quite often appear unhappy, withdrawn and antisocial. Because of the seeming hopelessness of their condition and the embarrassment of unsightly skin, such children frequently become loners and self-imposed exiles. In school they may be difficult to manage, constantly at odds with teacher and students alike, while at home they find it difficult to get along with other family members. These young people need all the assurance and support they can get from everyone in their vicinity: parents, siblings, friends, teachers and physician.

It is not unusual for school-age children who developed their atopic dermatitis during infancy to "outgrow" their skin symptoms. That's the good news. The bad news is that a sizable number of these youngsters will go on to develop hay fever and/or asthma symptoms.

Adolescent and adult stage   By the time a youngster has reached adolescence, quite often the eczema of the early childhood years has disappeared. If it has continued into the teenage years or begins at this time of life, the skin lesions tend to be of the dry, lichenified variety. The rash will mainly be found on the inside surface of the arms and legs as well as the wrists and hands. A rash present at this time will probably continue to some extent into the adult years.

The Role of Foods in Atopic Dermatitis

Many studies suggest that during the first six months of life, avoidance of potentially allergenic foods such as milk, eggs and wheat is helpful in retarding the development of atopic dermatitis. Of these foods, milk is by far the most likely to cause trouble. At the onset of symptoms, try replacing it with a nondairy formula. Soybean preparations such as Soyalac and Isomil or non-dairy preparations such as meat-base or lamb-base formulas are all possible substitutes. Breast feeding, a trend increasing among American mothers, is believed to be an aid in decreasing the risk of developing allergy conditions, especially in children with a hereditary predisposition.

While it is often difficult to pinpoint the specific foods that cause trouble, there is no question that food allergy plays a definite role in atopic dermatitis. If you have any suspicions in this direction, it would be wise to use a milk substitute and eliminate all suspected foods from the diet. Dietary regulation is one of the most important methods we have for both determining the cause and treating the symptoms of atopic dermatitis. Before making any major changes in your child's diet, however, always speak to your pediatrician. A well-balanced diet must be the foundation of any nutritional program.

Distinguishing Atopic Dermatitis from Other Skin Disorders

A number of skin conditions cause a rash that may be confused with atopic dermatitis. A brief description of these look-alikes follows.

Seborrheic dermatitis The table below will provide you with a comparison of these two common skin problems of early infancy.

Diaper rash This frequently irritating, itchy rash is limited exclusively

	Seborrheic Dermatitis	Atopic Dermatitis
Type of rash	Salmon-colored Greasy scales Clearly outlined	Reddened localized in single dry patches or generalized. Rash often is weeping and bloody because of constant scratching
Distribution of rash	Begins in scalp and progresses downwards. Facial involvement is usually partial. Found on neck, under the arms, on lower abdomen and genital regions	Found commonly on the face, mainly the cheeks. The neck, sometimes the scalp, the arms, legs and trunk
Itch	Rarely present	Most important symptom
Onset	Usually within the first two months of life	Generally after the age of two months
Family history of allergy	Usually absent	Usually present

to the diaper area. It is a result of a yeast or fungus infection or an irritation from ammonia, a normal component of urine. This condition responds quite well to appropriate topical treatment and frequent diaper changes.

Contact dermatitis   While it is true that there is a great deal of itching associated with contact dermatitis, the rash is usually localized to one area of the body. Treatment with a cortisone-containing cream or ointment usually eliminates the problem. The condition is caused by sensitivity to a variety of chemicals ranging from poison ivy to penicillin. Unlike atopic dermatitis, the rash is produced *exclusively* by sensitivity to things outside the body.

Tinea dermatitis   This condition is caused by a variety of different fungal agents. The lesions can in some situations be confused with atopic dermatitis. The best-known form is tinea pedis, commonly called athlete's foot. Other examples of this condition are tinea capitis, ringworm of the scalp, and tinea circinata, ringworm involving the face, neck and arms.

The rash caused by this fungus is usually a solitary, circular lesion with sharply outlined borders. On the scalp the lesion will produce a circumscribed local area of hair loss. The specific diagnosis is made by looking at scrapings from the lesions under a microscope. There are effective oral and topical medicines for this condition.

Pityriasis rosea   The typical appearance of pityriasis consists of slightly raised, salmon-colored lesions on the trunk. The rash can vary in shade from pale yellow to light red. The condition usually begins with a quarter- to half-dollar-sized lesion on the chest or back called the herald patch. Unlike atopic dermatitis, pityriasis rarely has any itching associated with it. It is a self-limiting condition, which means that it will clear up by itself within four to eight weeks.

Possible Complications of Atopic Dermatitis

Perhaps surprisingly, there are two rare but potentially life-threatening complications that can occur in a child with atopic dermatitis. One of them, eczema vaccinatum, has become considerably less of a problem since routine smallpox vaccinations have been discontinued. In brief, contact with smallpox vaccine or with individuals who have been vaccinated can produce smallpox-like lesions in a child with atopic dermatitis. Any person with atopic dermatitis should *never* be exposed to anyone who has recently been vaccinated for smallpox.

The other potentially severe condition is called either eczema herpeticum or Kaposi's varicelliform eruption. Exposure to and infection with the virus herpes simplex, which is responsible for cold sores, is the cause of this problem. The rash that develops looks like chicken pox and is found mainly on the face and those parts of the body where atopic dermatitis is active.

If there are large open skin areas which are weeping, then secondary bacterial infection and major problems caused by the loss of fluids and essential minerals can develop. A child with this condition may require admission to the hospital for supportive therapy.

Today I can still remember an eight-year-old boy named Carl who had chronic atopic dermatitis. For several hours one afternoon he had been in close contact with a friend who had several cold sores on his lip. Within a few days Carl was admitted to the hospital with severe eczema herpeticum. For seventy-two hours his temperature ranged between 104 and 106 degrees, and despite the latest in cooling techniques, antipyretic drugs and round-the-clock nursing, we were unable to break the fever. Finally, on the fourth hospital day, as I was becoming convinced the boy would surely die, his fever began to fall and his skin lesions started to dry. From then on his recovery was slow but regular. Today, it might be added, at age twenty-three, Carl is a six-foot-three giant, with, among many other personal assets, perfect skin. Even in the worst of medical situations, a positive outcome is possible.

Lesser but still significant complications can also result. Children with atopic dermatitis are at increased risk of developing superficial staph and strep skin infections. Such problems must be carefully watched for and aggressively treated with appropriate antibiotics if they appear. Any child with atopic dermatitis who begins complaining of difficulty in seeing or blurred vision must be examined by an eye doctor for the possible presence of atopic cataracts. This is a very rare complication involving the lens of the eye that can have a harmful effect on a child's vision. A brief examination by the doctor can determine whether a cataract is present.

One possible cause for this problem may be the prolonged use of oral cortisone drugs. Any child who must take this medicine for a long time should be checked at least once a year by an ophthalmologist.

Laboratory Evaluation

As a rule, the diagnosis of atopic dermatitis is made on the basis of a complete history and a thorough physical examination. The laboratory, unfortunately, can provide your doctor with relatively little assistance when it comes to this condition.

The IgE level, which is selectively elevated in allergic patients, is abnormally high in almost 100 percent of children with atopic dermatitis.

Most children with atopic dermatitis have highly irritable skin and are therefore poor candidates for direct allergy skin tests. I also have not been very impressed with the information obtained from skin testing children with eczema. If a youngster with atopic dermatitis has no symptoms of rhinitis or asthma, I generally do not recommend skin testing. On rare occasions a RAST test has been helpful in pinpointing specific causes for a child's eczema.

In the final analysis, perhaps the most effective testing and treatment approach to eczema is simply environmental control. Eliminate substances from your home that tend to cause allergic symptoms such as wool, feathers, dust and animal dander. For the younger child, dietary manipulation with the removal and reintroduction of certain groups of foods can be especially helpful (see the chapter on food allergies for more details regarding diet control).

A four-month-old named Robert was brought to my office with a suspicious-looking rash on his cheeks and ears. Robert had been placed on a milk-based formula on which he had thrived since birth. I ordered the formula suspended for ten days and substituted a soy-based preparation. Within the week the rash entirely disappeared. We next reintroduced the milk formula to Robert's diet and the rash quickly returned. The soy-based formula was then tried again, with the same positive results, and the family was convinced. Milk was removed from Robert's diet for the next six months and he remained free of the rash. When milk was reintroduced into his diet, Robert had no skin problems of any kind; his sensitivity had entirely disappeared.

This same method of dietary manipulation can be used with older atopic dermatitis children by removing a specific food or food group from the diet and observing the results. To date this technique is the most effective one we have of establishing a causal relationship between specific foods and atopic dermatitis.

Home Care for a Child with Atopic Dermatitis

General measures   There are a number of useful things parents can do to decrease and control the symptoms of atopic dermatitis.

When indoor air is dry, use a humidifier to increase the relative humidity to 40 to 45 percent. The increased moisture in the air will decrease skin irritation and itchiness, especially during the winter when the household atmosphere tends to be dry. While there are many types of humidifiers on the market, an ultrasonic cool mist humidifier in my opinion is the best. More on this below.

Children with eczema should avoid direct contact with obvious allergens, especially wool, feathers, furs and animal dander.

Certain foods with a high potential for causing allergic symptoms—such as milk, eggs and wheat—should be removed for a trial period from the diet of eczematous children. Whatever beneficial changes are going to take place should be evident after seven to fourteen days of avoidance.

Since emotional stress may intensify symptoms of atopic dermatitis, keep the child on an even keel and guide him away from particularly stressful situations. I realize it is easier in today's rather complicated world to make this recommendation than to carry it out, but even small efforts sometimes yield big results. Give it a try.

Control of itching   This is probably the single most important management area in the treatment of a child with atopic dermatitis. If the itch-scratch-itch-scratch cycle is interrupted, the skin lesions will tend to heal on their own. Unfortunately there is no uniformly effective anti-itch medication on the market today, and what works for one child fails with another. The drugs which have the best track records in my experience include the following:

> *Benadryl*   In addition to its anti-itch effects, this tried-and-true drug has a sedative action that is particularly desirable at bedtime—by the way, the time of day when scratching activity reaches its peak for most children. Benadryl is usually given three or four times a day. Consult your physician or pharmacist concerning the appropriate dose.
>
> *Atarax*   This is one of the most effective antihistamines for the control of itching. The starting dose usually is 1 milligram per pound a day. The dose may be increased every three to four days until the itch abates.
>
> *Periactin*   For some children this is quite effective. The dose is 0.1 milligram per pound a day divided in two or three doses.

As effective as antihistamines are when taken orally, these drugs should *never* be applied directly to the skin in a topical preparation; they have the potential to sensitize the skin and produce contact dermatitis.

Keep the skin moist.   In addition to using antihistamines for the control of itching, local skin care measures play a significant role in the overall management of atopic dermatitis. Well-moistened skin is less likely to itch.

The main purpose of skin moistener/lubricant preparations is to retain water within the superficial layers of the skin. One of the least expensive and most accessible of these lubricants is vegetable shortening. The problem, of course, with using preparations such as Crisco or Spry is their greasy feeling, but if they can be tolerated, these products are effective lubricants.

Some moisturizers, lubricants or emollients, whether available by prescription or over the counter, contain chemicals which may be irritating rather than soothing for some patients. Examples include paraben, a potential cause of contact dermatitis, and lanolin, a possible problem for children with a strong allergy to wool (lanolin is derived from sheep). Table 13 lists the frequently prescribed lubricants and shows what they contain.

Humidification   As mentioned, when the air in a room lacks adequate moisture it causes the skin to become dry and increases its potential for itching. The addition of water vapor to the household atmosphere via electronic humidifiers or by placing pans of water near the heat source in different rooms is a simple and effective way of approaching the situation. In order of increasing efficiency, the following methods will all improve the relative humidity level in your home:

Place pans of water near various heat sources throughout your home, near the radiators, steam pipes, stove.

Table 13. **Moisturizing Preparations**

Product Name	Contains Petrolatum	Contains Paraben	Contains Lanolin	Contains Urea
Acid Mantle				
cream	—	—	—	—
lotion	—	—	—	—
Aquacare				
cream	Yes	No	Yes	Yes
lotion	Yes	No	Yes	Yes
Aquaphor				
ointment	Yes	No	No	No
Carmol				
cream	No	No	No	Yes
lotion	No	No	No	Yes
Cetaphil	No	Yes	No	No
Eucerin				
ointment	Yes	No	No	Yes
Keri				
cream	No	No	Yes	Yes
lotion	No	No	Yes	Yes
Lubriderm				
lotion	Yes	No	Yes	Yes
Neutrogena				
cream	No	Yes	No	No
lotion	No	Yes	No	Yes

Set up a cool air vapor humidifier in the child's room and, if possible, in other rooms of the house.

Purchase an ultrasonic cool mist humidifier. Available at most appliance stores, this marvelous machine employs sound waves to break up water into a very fine vapor. The particles released by the mechanism then remain suspended in the air instead of condensing into pockets of moisture on the walls, furniture and floors, as happens with many cool air vapor humidifiers.

The major problem with ultrasonic mist humidifiers is their rather high cost—prices can range from $50 to $150. One consolation is that since the machine is being used for medical purposes, the cost can be deducted. Since the demand for these useful appliances is steadily increasing, it is likely that competition will soon bring their cost within the reach of most pocketbooks. Look for them in the off-season—at the end of winter—for the best buys.

Finally, the optimal relative humidity level for comfort is in the range of 40 to 45 percent. A household device called a humidistat will record this figure in much the same way a thermometer tells the room temperature, and it is well worth acquiring. Regardless of the method used to control the water content indoors, however, relative humidity must always be kept at an optimum level without major fluctuations. If carefully monitored, this can save your child many hours of discomfort.

General skin care measures

Bathing The question of whether taking a bath or shower is harmful or beneficial for eczematous patients is much debated. My own feeling is that during the colder months of the year when children with eczema seem to be most uncomfortable, they should be bathed briefly three or four times a week. Be sure to keep the water in these baths lukewarm, for as the water temperature rises it causes the superficial blood vessels to dilate or open and the surface temperature of the skin to increase, adding to the likelihood of increased itching. The use of bath oils such as Alpha-Keri will also help by retaining moisture within the superficial layers of the skin. Another commercial product with a similar effect is Aveeno, a natural oatmeal derivative that soothes and cleanses the skin.

As for skin cleansers, I have found that Dove soap is well tolerated by most children, perhaps because it contains a soothing cold cream base. Soaps that contain deodorants or perfume should be avoided. Simple soaps like Ivory and Camay are better, while special preparations such as Basis, Neutrogena and Lowila may be recommended by your doctor.

For children who cannot tolerate even occasional lukewarm baths, a commercial fat-free skin cleanser called Cetaphil is available, especially for very young children. Most pharmacies carry special hypoallergenic soaps with a pH level balanced for allergic children. Consult your physician for the one best suited to your child's condition. In general, use as little soap as possible on the child with atopic dermatitis and give baths only when they are absolutely necessary.

Indoor temperature The temperature in your home should be kept between 68 and 70 degrees. This is warm enough to keep children comfortable but not so hot that it makes them sweat (as mentioned previously, sweating aggravates skin irritation, which causes increased itching). During the summer, air conditioning can be used to maintain household temperatures at a comfortable level.

Nail care   One sharp or jagged fingernail can destroy days of a careful skin care regimen. Always keep nails short. When you trim, I suggest you avoid scissors or nail clippers that often leave small sharp edges. An emery board or nail file will get the job done and will provide perfectly smooth nails. Once a day quickly look at your child's fingernails. The old saying about an ounce of prevention is very appropriate in this situation. When it is practical, the use of cotton gloves on your child's hands at bedtime may limit the damage from nocturnal scratching.

Type of clothing   Loose-weave cottons are your best bet. When in contact with the skin these garments are very comfortable. Wool and various synthetic fibers are potentially irritating and should be avoided. Does this mean your child cannot wear a warm woolen winter coat when the thermometer plummets? Most of the time woolen outer garments are perfectly fine, and a cotton scarf worn around the neck will eliminate irritation caused by wool collars. As a rule of thumb, a child who has atopic dermatitis should wear clothing that is loose and comfortable, allowing plenty of circulation with a minimum of binding.

Medical Care

Several drugs are currently available for treating children with atopic dermatitis:

Topical cortisone   For many years cortisone creams, ointments and lotions have been the most important drugs used for the treatment of eczematous skin conditions. If a rash is scaly, dry and itchy, it will probably respond very well to these powerful anti-inflammatory preparations. Of course any time a steroid drug is prescribed, the doctor must consider the possible undesirable side effects from using the medication. Fortunately, when it comes to topical forms of cortisone the potential dangers are extremely small. You would literally have to dip your child into a vat of cortisone cream several times a day for many weeks before severe side effects from cortisone would develop.

Apply topical steroids only to those skin areas with a visible rash. Depending on the appearance of the rash your doctor will prescribe the appropriate form of topical steroid.

Small amounts of topical steroids should be applied to the rash three to four times a day. When the skin begins to clear, the frequency can be decreased and use of the drug eventually discontinued. One very important rule for parents to follow in the treatment of atopic dermatitis is to be aggressive, not to let the rash get ahead of you: it is always harder to play catch-up than to stay ahead of the game. Even when the rash is under control and the steroid agents are discontinued, always be ready to treat any recurrence vigorously. Here is a list of commonly used steroid preparations.

Topical Steroid Preparations

Low Potency	Concentration, in percentage	Intermediate Potency	Concentration, in percentage	High Potency	Concentration, in percentage
Aeroseb-HC aerosol	0.5	Aristocort-A	0.1	Aristocort-A cream, ointment	0.5
Aristocort-A cream, ointment	0.025	Cordran ointment, lotion	0.025 0.05	Diprosone cream, lotion, ointment	0.05
Cortaid cream, lotion, ointment, spray	0.05	Halog cream, ointment, solution	0.025	Diprosone aerosol	0.1
Cort-Dome cream, lotion	0.125 0.25 0.5 1.0	Kenalog cream, lotion, ointment	0.1	Halog cream, ointment, solution	0.1
Decaspray Aerosol	0.04	Kenalog-H cream	0.1	Halog-E cream	0.1
Dermacort cream & lotion	1.0	Kenalog spray	0.2	Kenalog cream, lotion, ointment	0.5

Topical Steroid Preparations (Continued)

Low Potency	Concentration, in percentage	Intermediate Potency	Concentration, in percentage	High Potency	Concentration, in percentage
Dermolate cream, ointment, spray, lotion	0.5	Synalar ointment, cream	0.025	Lidex cream, gel, ointment, solution	0.05
Hytone cream, lotion, ointment	2.5	Synemol cream	0.025	Lidex E cream	0.05
Kenalog cream, lotion, ointment	0.025	Tridesilon cream, ointment	0.05	Synalar-HP cream	0.2
Medrol topical	0.25 1.0	Valisone cream, lotion, ointment	0.1	Topicort cream, ointment	0.25
Synacort cream	1.0 2.5	Westcort cream, ointment	0.2	Topicort gel	0.05
Synalar cream	0.01			Topsyn	0.05
Synalar solution	0.01				
Valisone cream	0.01				

One word of caution: eczematous areas on the face should be treated with only the mildest forms of cortisone; the more potent steroid compounds can cause thinning of the skin and acne. While hydrocortisone in a concentration of 0.5 or 1 percent is particularly appropriate in this case, your physician should be your ultimate guide for dose and prescription.

What about orally administered steroids? The use of these drugs is usually recommended only if the atopic dermatitis cannot be controlled by any other measure, either antihistamine use, diet regulation and/or application of topical steroid agents. Once again, a word of caution: the results of orally administered cortisone are dramatic and the drugs are highly effective, but problems arise concerning the question of how long the medicine should be given. If the drug is administered over a short time and then discontinued abruptly, most patients will experience a rapid relapse and may be worse off than before the cortisone was taken; the dosage *must* be tapered off slowly. If, on the other hand, the medication is given for long periods of time, unwanted and sometimes dangerous side effects may occur. For these reasons the long-term use of oral steroids for atopic dermatitis should *rarely if ever* be prescribed.

Compresses   For acute symptoms of atopic dermatitis, especially lesions that are oozing and wet, compresses will soothe the irritation and dry the rash. These compresses can be made from cool water or Burrow's solution (aluminum acetate).

Compresses are quite effective for cleaning the rash and decreasing local itching. They cause fluids to evaporate and hence cool the wound, making it decidedly more comfortable for the child. Make a compress and apply it directly to the rash for ten to fifteen minutes, two to four times a day. When the acute symptoms have cleared, discontinue treatment.

Antibiotics   Quite frequently children with atopic dermatitis develop bacterial skin infections. You as parents must realize that this complication can occur and must be treated promptly with appropriate antibiotics. These infections develop most often on the arms and legs. The first indication of the presence of an infection is enlarged and sensitive lymph glands under the arms or in the groin. Any areas that are draining or appear to be very red are almost certainly infected. This complication develops because the skin surface has been broken by your child's prolonged scratching. Bacteria that are harmless on intact skin are able to get past the protective outer surface of the skin and cause an infection within the deeper layers.

Once the infection has been controlled, the eczematous rash will respond to treatment with topical steroids, lubricants and oral antihistamines. Parents should never use an antibiotic without first speaking with the doctor.

Immunotherapy   In my opinion, "allergy shots" are ineffective for the treatment of a child whose only "allergic" problem is atopic dermatitis. There certainly are youngsters who have allergic rhinitis or pollen asthma in addition to eczema. In this situation, immunotherapy would be indicated as treatment for the nasal and chest conditions. But if a doctor recommends immunotherapy just to treat a child's eczema, I would advise you to get a second opinion.

Diet If you are suspicious that a specific food or food family is causing your child's rash, eliminate the suspected offender for two weeks and see if the rash improves. If you are certain that positive changes have taken place, then that food should be eliminated from the diet for a three-to-six-month period. Cautious reintroduction of the food can then be tried to determine if the sensitivity still exists. In some cases the problem will be entirely gone and the child can return to her usual eating pattern.

Whether to perform allergy food tests remains an unanswered question. Some allergists claim that food testing is very important in the evaluation of a child with atopic dermatitis. In general, I have not found that doing these tests has helped me in the management of these youngsters. I still rely very heavily on an accurate, detailed food history and elimination diets in attempting to determine if specific foods are playing a role in a child's atopic dermatitis.

Contact Dermatitis

As the name implies, contact dermatitis is typified by skin eruptions resulting from direct contact with a variety of substances, most commonly household products, chemical compounds and plant materials. The rash begins at the point of direct contact and in general tends to remain localized. However, if exposure to the causative agent is repeated, there is a very good chance that the rash will spread. Unlike atopic dermatitis, a contact sensitivity is caused only by substances *external* to the body.

The condition appears in three main forms: allergic contact dermatitis, irritant contact dermatitis and photoallergic contact dermatitis.

Allergic contact dermatitis Children develop this condition after being exposed to a specific chemical, becoming sensitized to it, and developing a rash on subsequent exposure. The resulting dermatitis may be swollen, reddened, blistery or scaly. Itching is a constant symptom. An extremely common example is the rash produced by poison ivy, poison oak or poison sumac. Other causes might include hair dyes and rarely a sensitivity to airborne allergens.

Irritant contact dermatitis Here the substance causing the dermatitis is either a potent irritant such as a strong acid or a chemical substance. Diaper rash in infants, caused by metabolic breakdown substances in the stool and urine, is a classic example. People who frequently wash their hands with harsh soaps and detergents or those who come into continual contact with commercial chemicals such as cleaning fluids and paints are likewise prime candidates for this form of eczema.

Photoallergic contact dermatitis Two ingredients are essential to produce this condition: a specific chemical sensitizer and exposure to ultraviolet light. Neither alone will produce the rash; only their interaction will set the reaction in motion. As a rule, patients with photoallergic sensitivity are urged to stay out of the sun and to use sunscreen agents. Photoallergic contact dermatitis is the rarest form of contact dermatitis, especially among children.

Causes of Contact Dermatitis

Many of the ordinary chemical compounds used every day can cause contact dermatitis. A definitive list would take up pages. Some representative examples include:

antibiotic creams	leather products
antiperspirants	nail polish
baby oils	paints
bubble bath	perfumes
chromium salts	rubber products
cosmetics	shampoos
fabric dyes	soap
glues	solvents
hair dyes	synthetic fabrics
insecticides	topical anesthetics
jewelry	turpentine

It is of course virtually impossible to escape from all the potentially allergenic chemicals that have become so integral a part of our daily lives, and both parents and children can drive themselves mad by attempting such a thing. On the other hand, ordinary observation and common sense will take one a long way.

For instance, clues concerning the possible cause of contact dermatitis can be derived by noting the parts of the child's body where the dermatitis is located. If a child develops a rash on her neck, suspicion should be focused on her jewelry; metals in contact with the skin are a frequent cause of contact dermatitis. An outbreak on the wrist may be traced to a watchband or bracelet, and so on. By careful observation, you may be able to identify the substance or substances responsible for the problem.

Poison ivy   One of the most conspicuous of these potentially avoidable substances is poison ivy. The seriousness of this condition can run the gamut from a mild nuisance to a major medical problem that requires hospital admission. The source of the trouble is the sap from the leaves and stem of the *Rhus radicans* plant. Once you have become sensitized by contact with the sap, subsequent exposure will cause the appearance of a blistery, highly itchy rash that can literally drive you out of your skin.

Laura was sent to me by another physician for an unsolvable problem, a "mysterious" rash that had been spreading steadily for a week and was uncontrollable by means of the usual over-the-counter salves and ointments. By the time I examined the fretful child, the rash covered her entire body from head to toe. No one had considered poison ivy and with good reason: it was the middle of January.

In reviewing Laura's history I learned that the family owned a frisky German shepherd that was allowed to run free in the woods behind their house. When the dog returned from his peregrinations, it was Laura's job to fetch a towel and wipe him dry. It turned out the dog enjoyed romping through parts of the woods where the dried stems of last summer's poison ivy crop still stood, and in so doing he had gotten poison ivy sap on his coat. Naturally, when Laura toweled him dry the sap rubbed off onto her hands, and there was the answer. Treatment with cortisone brought the rash quickly under control, and within ten days Laura's skin was clear.

One point of this case history to bear in mind is that oral cortisone is the medicine of choice for severe poison ivy. Treatment must sometimes be continued for up to three weeks for particularly bad cases, but in the end cortisone will eliminate the condition. Also helpful is calamine lotion or calamine with phenol, but only if the poison ivy is mild and limited in one part of the body. There is a lotion on the market which contains both calamine lotion and the antihistamine Benadryl, Caladryl; as I mentioned earlier, topical antihistamines are potent sensitizers and I would not recommend any preparation that contains them. For localized poison ivy, cortisone cream should be sufficient to control the rash.

The same holds true for desensitization/immunotherapy treatment for poison ivy: I do not recommend it. This procedure calls for a series of regular injections or for the administration of drops of poison ivy extract placed under the tongue. Though from time to time doctors have claimed success with these measures, my own judgment and that of most other allergists is that they are not effective. There is no scientific evidence to prove that this treatment works!

What other symptomatic treatment is useful for poison ivy? For the itching, cool baths are temporarily soothing and will make the patient feel more comfortable and relaxed. Be careful that your child's fingernails are well clipped, for too much scratching, as with atopic dermatitis, can introduce bacteria into the inner layers of the skin and promote bacterial infections. Oral antihistamines such as Benadryl, Atarax and Periactin can also be useful in decreasing intensive itching, and I often prescribe them. Once again, remember that the application of topical antihistamines may cause sensitization and produce an allergic rash on top of the poison ivy. They should not be used.

All in all, though poison ivy is a highly annoying and uncomfortable condition, with prompt recognition and appropriate therapy this common example of contact dermatitis can be kept well controlled.

Evaluation and Treatment of Allergic Contact Dermatitis

Evaluation As in all allergic conditions, a detailed history and thorough examination are essential steps in the evaluation of any patient with contact dermatitis. If the physician suspects that the dermatitis is of the allergic variety, he may then recommend patch testing to determine which substances are causing the problem (see page 28).

Patch testing will be performed after the acute outbreak has been brought under control by appropriate treatment. The patch itself is composed of a soft cloth or paper impregnated with a specific allergen and placed on the upper arm or upper portion of the back. Over it an adhesive bandage type dressing is fitted and the patch area is allowed to incubate for forty-eight hours. (If intense local itching appears before this time, it indicates a high degree of sensitivity. The doctor should be notified right away and the test discontinued.)

Once the forty-eight hours have passed, the patches are removed. The test sites are examined within two to four hours and then examined again two days later. A positive reaction consists of redness, local swelling and blisters at the test site. Once the positive substances are identified, avoiding them will ordinarily prevent recurrence of the rash.

Treatment   The rash caused by contact dermatitis is treated in much the same manner as atopic dermatitis. Cool compresses are useful for soothing a weeping rash, and topical steroid creams or ointments will keep most lesions under control. Occasionally, appropriate short doses of oral cortisone will be given for particularly stubborn or severe cases. The skin care and itch control procedures mentioned earlier for atopic dermatitis are equally appropriate for the control of contact dermatitis.

Fortunately, most cases of contact dermatitis can be diagnosed and subsequently treated. Avoidance of the substance responsible for the problem will "cure" the condition. There are rarely any permanent skin changes as the result of contact dermatitis.

Questions and Answers About Eczema

Is aspirin ever used to control severe itching associated with atopic dermatitis?

There is clinical evidence that some children respond well to aspirin, for the control of persistent itching. If you cannot relieve your child's itching with antihistamines, then aspirin is worth a try.

What effect, if any, does being outdoors in sunny weather have on a child's atopic dermatitis?

During the warmer months of the year many children with atopic dermatitis tend to benefit from being outdoors. Exposure to sunlight decreases the intensity of eczematous rashes, and for some children the sun appears to have an almost miraculous effect; their skin becomes less dry and itching decreases dramatically. The seashore is especially therapeutic in this regard, and for the majority of young sufferers the blend of saltwater and sunlight has a wonderfully healing influence.

Is eczema ever contagious?

Though the characteristic rash it produces certainly has a menacing appearance, eczema is in no way contagious and one child cannot under any circumstances "catch" it from another. The only time contagion becomes an issue is when a secondary infection accompanies the eczema, and even then it is the infection that spreads, not the atopic dermatitis.

Once eczema has disappeared, will the child continue to have dry skin into adult life?

The tendency toward a dry skin condition is something you are usually born with. I would say that your particular skin characteristics, whether oily or dry, persist throughout life.

What happens to the eczematous child when she develops a viral infection such as a cold or flu?

In my experience a viral infection will generally tend to aggravate the rash in a child with atopic dermatitis. However, on rare occasions I have also seen patients who for some inexplicable reason have *fewer* skin symptoms and complaints at this time.

What role do emotions play in the life of a child with atopic dermatitis?

Any time you are dealing with a chronic medical condition such as atopic dermatitis, the emotions must invariably be considered. Frustration, anxiety and anger all tend to aggravate the child's condition and make the rash significantly worse. For some children it may even be necessary to consider a mild tranquilizer, I rarely have had to prescribe such drugs. Sometimes I recommend that the parent take the tranquilizer so that he or she can cope with the severely eczematous child. Certainly a calm, stable atmosphere in the home is a worthy goal to aim for that will exert a definite and undeniably therapeutic effect on most children.

Allergies of the Ear and Eye

Allergic Conditions of the Ear

A three-year-old named Leslie was recently brought to my office for an allergy evaluation. Leslie's chief problems, her parents explained to me, were her inability to get along with her nursery school classmates and poor language development. In reviewing Leslie's medical history I found that she had been suffering with recurring ear infections that required frequent antibiotic treatment. After repeated episodes of this condition, Leslie's pediatrician began to suspect that there might be an underlying allergic problem, so she was referred to me.

Leslie's physical examination revealed that there was fluid trapped behind her eardrum in the middle ear. A subsequent hearing test gave evidence of a low-grade hearing loss in both ears. Leslie, it seemed, had a condition known as serous otitis, or more technically, otitis media with effusion (OME). The decrease of hearing that resulted from the fluid accumulation was clearly interfering with both her language development and her ability to relate to her classmates.

In an attempt to get rid of the accumulated fluid a variety of antihistamines and decongestants were prescribed. Unfortunately, Leslie had only a partial response to the medicines and finally had to have the fluid drained from the middle ear by a procedure known as a myringotomy. A tiny incision is made in the eardrum (tympanic membrane) and the usually thickened fluid is removed by a suction machine. Drainage tubes (tympanostomy tubes) are then left in place to make sure that the fluid doesn't reaccumulate. These tubes can remain in place and function well for twelve to eighteen months; they can then be easily removed by an ear, nose and throat doctor. In Leslie's case, within two weeks, according to her parents and her nursery school teacher, she was "an entirely new child." All symptoms, both physical and psychological, had disappeared.

This made us all proud, of course, but nothing had really been wrong with this bright child's developmental and emotional skills from the start. She had been suffering from a low-grade hearing loss, and because of this, her inability to communicate with the outside world made her angry, frustrated and handicapped.

Leslie's story illustrates an important point, that a physical problem can have a significant social and psychological impact on a person's life. Parents and physicians should consider possible unrecognized problems involving the eyes and ears in the case of any child not progressing normally at home and in school. The insidious thing about such conditions is that parents are not ordinarily trained to recognize their symptoms and, of course, the child is too young to verbalize them and may be unaware of them, too. In this chapter we will examine a number of ear and eye ailments, both to provide parents with criteria for identifying them and as an aid for both parent and child to deal with them.

Before getting into the hows and whys of childhood hearing loss problems, let's take a look at the anatomy of the ear and get a quick overview of how it functions. The human ear is divided into external, middle and inner sections.

The external ear   This is the shell-shaped part of the ear visible from the outside. It consists of the auricle, which collects air vibrations resulting from sounds in the environment, and the auditory canal, which transmits these vibrations to the middle ear.

The middle ear, or tympanum   This section is normally filled with air. It houses the eardrum (tympanic membrane) and is connected to the nasopharynx at the back of the throat by means of the eustachian tube. Within its depths, as can be seen in Figure 9, there is a chain of three small moveable

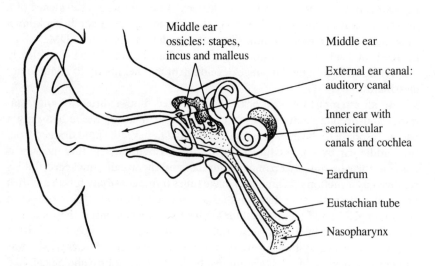

Cross section of a normal ear

bones called the stapes, incus and malleus. When air vibrations strike the eardrum, they set in motion these bones, which then transmit the vibrations to the inner ear.

The inner ear or labyrinth   In this final portion of the ear a linkup is made with the auditory nerve. This nerve then transmits these vibrations directly to the brain, where they are decoded and interpreted as specific sounds. The semicircular canals are involved in the equilibrium or balance mechanism of the body. The cochlea is a resonating chamber helping us to distinguish differences in sounds.

Allergic and Nonallergic Ear Problems: Telling Them Apart

Ordinarily the ear is a highly sensitive and receptive organ, and we take its functions for granted. Trouble begins when the mechanism is thrown out of balance by disease or by an allergic reaction. The most common of such problems is acute otitis media, or as it is known to parents far and wide, the dreaded earache. This condition is *not* allergic, and parents should note the differences between its symptoms and those of genuine allergic conditions:

Acute otitis media (AOM)   Just about all of us, young and old, have suffered from the pain of this common infection; in fact it is estimated that by age three, 70 percent of all children have suffered from AOM at least once. The highest incidence takes place between the ages of six and twenty-four months. Allergy is not the cause of this infectious condition, and a positive family or personal history of allergy will not increase your child's risk of developing otitis media.

The most common symptoms of acute otitis media are the sudden onset of severe ear pain usually associated with a fever. Occasionally a child suffering from this ailment will have neither of these signs, but such instances are an exception. Sometimes the ear feels hot to the touch and the child acts irritable and out of sorts. Occasionally the pain becomes so strong that the patient cries out and is inconsolable.

Otitis media is classified as acute if the symptoms clear up within three weeks, chronic if it lasts twelve weeks or more. Fluid accumulation in the middle ear—more on this below—may be associated with acute otitis media, though it is far more likely to occur when the condition is chronic.

Treatment with an appropriate antibiotic over a ten- to fourteen-day period will usually cure the problem. A small number of children do develop accumulation of fluid behind the eardrum during the healing phase of AOM. This accumulation of fluid in the middle ear is known as an effusion.

If the effusion remains for several weeks, it becomes concentrated and eventually takes on a gluelike consistency. When this occurs, there will almost certainly be some degree of hearing loss. If an effusion persists, it may be necessary to make a small incision (myringotomy) in the eardrum and drain the thickened fluid from the middle ear. Quite often drainage (tympanostomy) tubes will be left in the eardrum to prevent fluids from reaccumulating. For this procedure an overnight admission to the hospital may be necessary.

Parents should be on the lookout for any of the following situations that may indicate possible hearing loss due to an effusion in a child recovering from otitis media:

> the child continually increases the volume of the radio or record player.
> the child seems unable to hear people who are speaking at a normal conversational level.
> the child's grades suddenly take a dramatic turn for the worse.

If any of these situations are present, have your child's hearing checked. Most pediatricians are equipped to do screening hearing tests in their offices.

Secretory otitis media, or serous otitis   Unlike acute otitis media, serous otitis is sometimes linked to allergies and is prevalent in children who suffer from allergic rhinitis. The persistence of fluid in the middle ear may lead to hearing problems and must be treated aggressively. While there are no accurate statistics to indicate what percentage of children who develop serous otitis are actually allergic, an educated guess based on information published in medical journals tells us that approximately one-third have an underlying allergic predisposition.

What causes serous otitis? We know that a significant increase in the size of the adenoids can interfere with the normal drainage functions of the eustachian tubes, thus leading to fluid accumulation in the middle ear. The mechanism by which an allergic reaction in the nose leads to such middle ear effusion works roughly as follows: Swelling of the nasal mucous membranes extends into the region where the eustachian tube opens into the nasopharynx (see Figure 9). The mouth of the eustachian tube may become partially or completely blocked depending on the amount of allergic swelling in the area. This obstruction interferes with the normal drainage of ear fluid, which then becomes trapped in the middle ear cavity. When allergic symptoms are treated with antihistamines or decongestants, the swelling in the nose decreases and normal function of the eustachian tubes may be restored.

Symptoms of serous otitis revolve around hearing impairment, and, significantly, the fever and malaise found in AOM is not present. Since the effusion in serous otitis is usually nonirritating, large amounts of the fluid can sometimes accumulate without producing obvious symptoms. Common complaints consist of statements such as "My ears are blocked up," or "It sounds as if I'm hearing underwater," or "It feels like my ears are dripping." Rarely is pain associated with serous otitis unless an infection happens to be present as well.

When a child with this condition is brought to a physician's office and examined, the doctor will most likely see "bubbles" or even an actual fluid level located behind the eardrum. Occasionally the fluid will exert so much pressure that the child's eardrum bulges outward. Conservative treatment normally consists of decongestants or antihistamines, though I must tell you that several recent studies have questioned the effectiveness of these preparations, and prolonged accumulation of fluid usually requires either a simple drainage procedure (myringotomy) or the placement of drainage (tympanostomy) tubes in the ears.

Eustachian tube dysfunction   When the eustachian tube, which connects the inner ear to the nasopharynx, doesn't function properly, one result is the accumulation of fluid in the middle ear.

The normal functions of the eustachian tube are:

to equalize the pressure between the nose, throat (nasopharynx) and middle ear

to block nasopharyngeal secretions from reaching the middle ear

to properly ventilate and supply oxygen to the middle ear

to serve as the pathway for the fluid normally produced in the middle ear to drain into the throat

If the eustachian tube fails to function properly because of either a physical obstruction, such as a tumor (very rare) or what is termed abnormal potency, whereby the opening (ostium) of the eustachian tube (in the nasopharynx) either fails to close properly or opens at inappropriate times, there exists the possibility of developing an infection or the accumulation of fluid in the middle ear.

Specific conditions that can lead to eustachian tube dysfunction include the following:

unrepaired cleft palates in infants

submucous cleft palates

divided uvula (the fleshy mass of tissue suspended from the center of the soft palate over the back of the tongue)

tumors involving the middle ear

certain degenerative muscle disorders

Spotting Hearing Problems Early

Now to the heart of the matter: how to recognize the symptoms of a low-grade a hearing loss. What should you as a parent be on the lookout for in order to minimize the possibilities of this hazard?

During the first year of life a child who is unreasonably irritable, who sleeps poorly and who doesn't react appropriately to loud noises may be suffering from hearing impairment.

During the first two to three years, a delay in the development of normal speech patterns may be indicative of hearing difficulties.

In older children any of the following behavior patterns can be tipoffs to low-grade hearing difficulties:

slow language development
the need to have statements repeated several times
lack of attention and concentration
frequent disobedience
complaints of popping noises in the ear, dull earaches, or a sensation of
    fullness in the head
a tendency to turn the volume of the radio or TV up inordinately loud
a tendency to speak too loudly
an inability to hear the phone ring or to hear the voice on the other end
    when picking up
disobedience, disinterest and boredom in school; underachievement in
    general

If several of these symptoms are present simultaneously, it should alert parents to the possibility that something more than childish laziness or contrariness is at the heart of the matter. If you have suspicions, don't hesitate to bring your child to the doctor's office for a hearing evaluation.

To avoid the development of middle ear problems, never place infants into postures or positions that make it possible for them to aspirate fluid into the eustachian tube. Propping a bottle or using a poorly ventilated nipple are two situations that may lead to aspiration of fluid into the eustachian tube.

Undergoing a Hearing Evaluation Test

What procedures await your child when brought to the doctor's office for a hearing evaluation? First, as always, the doctor will review your child's personal and medical history. Then a physical examination will follow, focusing on the ears.

The doctor will examine your child's ears with a piece of equipment called a pneumatic otoscope. This is the standard otoscope to which a tube fitted with a rubber air bulb is attached. By squeezing the bulb when the otoscope is placed in the ear, air is forced against the tympanic membrane. This will cause the eardrum to move, and the doctor can tell if there is fluid behind the drum by the way it moves in response to the change in air pressure. The examination is called pneumatic otoscopy. The doctor may also place a vibrating tuning fork near the ear to check for hearing loss. A somewhat more sensitive method, designed to see how accurately the eardrum receives sound vibrations, is tympanometry. It is administered by means of a small apparatus called the tympanometer. The test is quick, painless and is especially valuable for evaluating the hearing of children six months or older. Of all the hearing tests given at the physician's office, the most accurate is called audiometry. This procedure is generally administered to children over five years of age. It is carried out in a quiet room where the child is required to indicate when he hears sounds of different wavelengths piped into his ears. The response to these sounds is then analyzed and evaluated, the result providing a highly accurate profile of the patient's ability to hear at a variety of sound levels. Occasionally an X-ray of a child's neck will be performed in order to check the size of the adenoids. If the adenoids become enlarged they may produce obstruction at the mouth of the eustachian tube, causing fluid to accumulate in the middle ear.

When fluid buildup in the middle ear is unresponsive to medical treatment, it will be necessary to remove the trapped secretions from behind the tympanic membrane. This is done by making a tiny incision in the eardrum, a procedure known as a myringotomy. The thickened secretions are then sucked out with a syringe, which relieves the pressure on the middle ear, and provides a specimen that can be sent for appropriate bacteriologic study. Occasionally this procedure will be performed in a doctor's office, though more commonly it is done in a hospital.

Treatment for Serous Otitis

Once the diagnosis of serous otitis has been made, environmental measures for the control of allergy such as those outlined throughout the book should be used for a child suffering from allergic ear problems. It is especially important to maintain adequate humidity in the child's immediate environment.

Now for specific treatment plans:

Antibiotics   If any evidence of bacterial infection appears either as general symptoms (fever, malaise) or during a physical and laboratory examination (a red, painful eardrum, a positive bacterial culture) a ten- to fourteen-day course of treatment with an appropriate antibiotic will be required.

Antihistamines/decongestants   There is no consensus among allergists regarding how effective these medications really are in relieving serous otitis. My own experience indicates that an antihistamine, a decongestant or a combination preparation can *in some cases* provide symptomatic relief. A wide variety of these drugs are available over the counter at any pharmacy. However, before starting your child on *any* course of treatment, please speak with a physician.

Topical decongestants and steroids   A word of caution here: the prolonged daily use of nonprescription nose drops and sprays such as Afrin, Otrivin, Neo-Synephrine and Privine (to name only a few) will *worsen,* not improve, both nasal and middle ear symptoms. Such medications should be used for no longer than three to five days at a time and then discontinued (for a more thorough discussion of this matter, see page 123). Cortisone nasal sprays (Nasalide, Beconase, Vancenase) are quite effective in reducing both swelling and inflammation in the nasal passageways. These preparations are poorly absorbed, highly surface-active forms of cortisone. This means that they work where they are sprayed (in the nose) and are rarely absorbed into the body. The likelihood that they will cause the types of undesirable side effects associated with prolonged oral use of cortisone is very, very small. Of course they should only be used as recommended by your doctor and only for as long as necessary.

Immunotherapy   The use of allergy injection therapy should be limited to that small group of children for whom a proven relationship between specific allergies and serous otitis can be documented. I recall having seen a five-year-old girl some years ago who, like clockwork, suffered from a hearing problem for four to six weeks every spring. When the youngster was tested for different allergens, positive results were found to tree and grass pollen. A course of decongestants and antihistamines was prescribed, but it was not effective, so she was started on a regular program of allergy shots. By the second season of treatment the girl's hearing problems had disappeared, and to date they have not returned. Notice, however, that in this case a definite cause-and-effect relationship between specific allergens and the serous otitis was established *before* immunotherapy began. Unless this relationship can be proven, such treatment is entirely inappropriate and should *not* be recommended. At the same time, patients who have proven allergic rhinitis as well as serous otitis are certainly potential candidates for immunotherapy.

Surgery   If the various medical treatments outlined so far fail to clear up middle ear problems caused by serous otitis, it may be necessary to consider surgical treatment.

Most common among such operations is the insertion of a small curved plastic or Teflon tube through the eardrum, the purpose being to drain secretions from behind the middle ear and to equalize the pressure on both sides of the eardrum. This surgical procedure, though a somewhat simple one, may require an overnight stay in the hospital. The tube implanted in the ear during the operation may remain in place for weeks, and more usually months, until all infection has disappeared and hearing is restored. The operation is known as a myringotomy with placement of tympanostomy tubes.

A second surgical procedure that may also be recommended is an adenoidectomy. If a child's adenoids become so enlarged that they cause compression of the mouth of the eustachian tube (with obstruction and a consequent buildup of fluids in the middle ear), then this operation is clearly indicated. One word of caution, however: there is no way to guarantee that the adenoids will not grow back after they have been removed.

Finally, it is very difficult for both the parent and the doctor to know exactly what course this condition will take in any given child. Will it resolve itself over a period of weeks and months without any treatment? Perhaps, but not always. What effect will a partial hearing loss have on the child's development years? We do not know. No doubt it will have *some* negative effect, but just how great will this effect be?

While none of these intangibles can be precisely measured, it is my feeling that during the childhood years *any evidence whatsoever* of hearing loss, no matter how slight, should be given immediate and vigorous treatment to insure against a potentially permanent handicap. Whenever the health of a primary sense organ is involved, none of us can ever afford to take a wait and see attitude.

Allergic Conditions of the Eyes

Alicia, aged six, becomes impossible to live with from the middle of August until some time in early October. Every morning she awakens with red, swollen eyes and an angry temperament to match. She constantly complains that her eyes are itching, and whenever she goes outdoors her eyes swell up. There is simply no relief from this burdensome routine until late fall.

Roger, an eleven-year-old, has had severe allergy symptoms during the spring and summer for several years. He regularly complains of an uncontrollable itching sensation around his eyes and the feeling that there are pebbles under his eyelids. He has become so sensitive to sunlight that whenever he goes outside he must wear dark glasses.

Cynthia, age thirteen, has suffered from severe atopic dermatitis since she was four. Over the past several months she has complained that the quality of her vision is becoming impaired. An examination at the ophthalmologist's office revealed early evidence of cataract formation.

Do you recognize any of these symptoms in your own child? Each has eye discomfort caused by allergic conditions. Alicia suffers from allergic conjunctivitis caused by ragweed sensitivity. Roger is a victim of vernal conjunctivitis. Cynthia's cataracts are a very unusual complication that can occur with severe atopic dermatitis. Of the three conditions, allergic conjunctivitis is the most prevalent, followed at a good distance by vernal conjunctivitis. Fortunately, cataracts resulting from atopic dermatitis are relatively rare.

Allergic conjunctivitis   This allergic eye disease is usually associated with allergic rhinitis. It may occur as an acute explosive reaction that involves either one or both eyes and can become a chronic problem.

The acute form produces sudden swelling of the conjunctiva (white portion of the eye) along with redness and profuse tearing. Frequently these children have an exquisite sensitivity to light (photophobia) and are extremely uncomfortable. They certainly require immediate medical attention.

The chronic form of allergic conjunctivitis is less likely to cause reddened, tearing eyes and more likely to produce eyes that are itchy and dry with blurred vision and increased light sensitivity. The white portion (conjunctiva) of the eye may have a finely granular or roughened appearance (if your child will let you close enough to take a look). Treatment for atopic conjunctivitis consists of both local and systemic medications. Vasoconstrictor eye drops containing such drugs as phenylepherine, tetrahydrozoline and naphazoline are highly effective in controlling both the acute and chronic forms and are frequently prescribed. Steroid-based ointments and drops are also effective for serious cases. Cortisone preparations may be of great benefit to patients suffering from eye ailments, but if they are used for long periods of time without careful medical supervision, *severe ophthalmic complications can result.* It is my feeling that an ophthalmologist should be involved *whenever* cortisone eye preparations are prescribed and that the patient should be *closely monitored* to insure that unacceptable side effects do not develop.

Oral antihistamines are commonly prescribed for allergic conjunctivitis (see page 122 for a discussion and Table 7 for a list of the most commonly used antihistamines). These drugs are readily available and have an excellent safety record in the treatment of this condition. Finally, the newest and perhaps most promising medication on the market is a 4-percent solution of cromolyn sodium (see page 86) called Opticrom. Like all forms of cromolyn, this drug works as a prophylactic agent, meaning that it is only effective if administered *before* eye symptoms develop. Side effects are almost nonexistent when the drug is used correctly; therefore, Opticrom can be taken for long periods of time.

Vernal conjunctivitis   This disorder is a relatively uncommon form of conjunctivitis that plagues sufferers in the spring and summer months. The exact cause is unknown. Children with vernal conjunctivitis complain of a severe itching involving both eyes and of the feeling that something is somehow "stuck" in their eyes. Frequently a doctor will diagnose this condition by inverting the child's upper eyelid and searching for a characteristic cobblestone appearance, an effect that appears exactly as the word describes: small, hard, stonelike bumps encrusted on the inner side of the upper eyelid. Blurred vision and extreme sensitivity to light round out this ailment's unpleasant list of symptoms. Many more males than females have this condition.

Even in extremely stubborn cases, vernal conjunctivitis fortunately tends to clear up by itself before a child becomes an adult. Topical steroids are the most effective medications for treating this frustrating condition, but their use must be *scrupulously monitored* by an eye doctor. Most other ophthalmic medications are simply not very effective in this situation and at best will produce temporary symptomatic relief.

Conjunctivitis associated with atopic dermatitis   The eyelids in this form of conjunctivitis may be thickened and very dry with a conspicuously "cracked" appearance. Occasionally there will be wet, weeping lesions. The itching associated with this condition is severe and persistent compared with the conjunctivitis that accompanies hay fever. The cobblestone lesions, seen on the inner surface of the upper eyelid in vernal conjunctivitis, may show up on the lower lid in the atopic variety. In severe cases the cornea can become involved with the production of ulcers and cataracts; fortunately these findings are rare. (A complaint of severe light sensitivity should alert you to the possibility that corneal involvement may be taking place.) If such symptoms persist, consult a doctor *immediately.*

Treatment with the Opticrom and topical steroids generally proves effective in symptom control.

Contact dermatitis is a condition that not infrequently involves the eye. In this situation, the eyelids rather than the conjunctiva are primarily attacked. As discussed in the contact dermatitis section, there are many possible causes for the development of this itchy, scaling rash. Not uncommonly, teenage girls have this problem because of sensitivity to either eye makeup or nail polish.

Treatment consists of avoidance of the sensitizing substance and the use of mild strength steroid creams applied carefully to the eyelids. As always, before using any medicine, call and at least discuss the situation with the doctor.

Questions and Answers About Ear and Eye Allergies

Can permanent damage be done to the ear after a myringotomy procedure?

A myringotomy consists of making a small incision in the tympanic membrane for the purpose of removing fluids trapped in the middle ear. The procedure is usually performed in a hospital, though it can also be done in a well-equipped otolaryngologist's (an ear, nose and throat specialist's) office. The incision heals easily and completely, and there should be no problems of any kind resulting from this procedure. Certainly, under normal conditions there will be no permanent damage of any kind.

After a drainage tube (tympanostomy) has been removed from the ear, will the hole heal completely?

In most cases the incision in the tympanic membrane made to accommodate a drainage tube will close spontaneously. In a very small number of cases, usually those in which the patient has suffered severe repeated ear infections over a prolonged period of time, the damage done to the eardrum by these infections may cause the hole to remain permanently open. Even if this situation develops, it does not pose a particularly serious problem and it rarely interferes with a child's ability to hear.

If chronic serous otitis remains untreated, will this create the possibility of hearing loss?

If fluid is allowed to remain trapped in the middle ear for long periods of time, I believe the potential for hearing damage certainly exists. What happens is that the fluid becomes progressively thicker so that eventually the child ends up with a condition known rather graphically as "glue ear." In this case a degree of hearing loss almost always results. With the proper treatment in most cases—either medical, surgical or both—the problem can be corrected.

What symptoms are most commonly associated with eye allergies?

Itching, tearing and redness of the eyes are the most characteristic ones. Dark circles under the eyes, the so-called allergic shiners, are also typical, both for children with nasal allergies and eye allergies. Whatever the case, always speak with your doctor if eye symptoms of any kind persist. Certain infections cause symptoms similar to those produced by allergy, but their treatment is quite different.

Can a child's sight be permanently damaged if the eyes become swollen shut during an allergic reaction?

Although a youngster who is unable to open his eyes owing to an allergic reaction may become quite terrified, rest assured there will be no residual visual impairment once the external swelling has responded to appropriate treatment. Such treatment normally consists of oral antihistamines, decongestant/antihistamine eye drops, and cold compresses applied to the swollen eyes. Cortisone drops can be very effective for this type of reaction.

The white portion of my child's eyes has become so swollen that it actually bulges out of the eyes. How dangerous is this situation?

The white portion of the eye, the conjunctiva, can become dramatically swollen after exposure to almost any allergen—for example, pollen or contact with a household pet such as a dog or cat. If such swelling occurs, the allergist should be contacted immediately. Treatment with an oral antihistamine, topical steroids and local vasoconstrictor eye drops will normally control the situation. There is almost no chance that permanent eye damage can result from such a reaction.

Parents Beware: Controversial Practices in the Field of Allergic Medicine

One of the questions I am frequently asked by parents is how the different tests and procedures used by allergists are actually developed, tested and made safe. My answer is that the techniques commonly used in the diagnosis and treatment of allergic conditions are accepted by the medical profession *only* after they have been scientifically proven to be effective. This method, I tell them, is the heart and soul of all good science, and is especially crucial to the development of all worthwhile advances in the field of medicine. Among its fundamental premises are the following concepts:

A procedure is valid only when its results can be consistently duplicated by individuals working independently of one another and all possibility that these results are due to coincidence, accident or placebo effect has been ruled out.

Final conclusions regarding the effectiveness of a specific diagnostic procedure or medical treatment program can be reached only after analyzing data from a large number of patients. This information must be statistically evaluated before recommendations are made to the medical profession and the general public.

Using these guidelines as the foundation of medical experimentation, enough clinical and laboratory experience has been accumulated through the years to provide allergists with a variety of effective diagnostic techniques and theraputic approaches for the management of allergic patients.

It would, of course, be immodest and incorrect for allergists to claim that their present methods for treating allergic diseases cannot be improved upon. They can, and they will be. What is most important to understand is that new procedures will be accepted by the mainstream of medical practitioners *only* after they have been *proven* to be safe and effective.

In practical terms this means that a physician in Stamford, Connecticut, using a certain procedure and a physician in Boise, Idaho, employing the same method will, under similar circumstances, obtain similar results. These doctors are in effect enjoying the benefits of the same principle, the principle of objective experimentation via the scientific method.

At the risk of sounding like a textbook writer for a moment, let's look a bit more closely at this notion of the scientific method, because I want you to gain at least a passing awareness of how this important principle works. Why? So that if in the future you see a physician who promises to clear up your child's allergic problem with a special diet or a new type of serum, you will be knowledgeable enough to ask the appropriate questions. If the doctor is unwilling to answer your questions, attempts to give you highly technical explanations or becomes evasive, you are probably in the wrong office!

Two main questions underlie the issue of medical legitimacy: How do medical research scientists determine that a laboratory procedure or new form of treatment is safe, reliable and effective? If we compare a traditional allergist and a physician who uses what might be called controversial practices, what differences might we find in the manner in which they evaluate new treatment methods or testing procedures?

First, a description of the classical approach. Without becoming too technical, a step-by-step description follows of what a research scientist must do concerning the definition, observation, testing, evaluation and description of a new medical technique before this procedure is accepted for general use by the medical community.

Hypothesis   The hypothesis represents the concept or idea behind the procedure. This concept may involve a notion for the development of a laboratory test or for a new method of treatment. The hypothesis should be clearly stated and based as fully as possible on previously established knowledge and information.

Procedures and test materials   The exact steps and materials necessary to perform the test must next be outlined very precisely. Such an outline will enable other technicians working anywhere in the world to duplicate the same test procedures.

Subjects   If the test requires patient participation, a specific description of the study group should accompany all information concerning technique and chemical reagents. This procedure permits other investigators to compare equal patient groups when evaluating the diagnostic or treatment procedure.

Test and control groups   When it is time to perform clinical trials of the new procedure, two groups of subjects approximately the same in size, age, sex and degree of illness are chosen, the first for actual testing, the second as a so-called control group. For example, if we are testing a new asthma medicine, the test group will be given a pill that actually contains the new medicine. The second group, the control group, will receive pills that look exactly like the actual medicine but which actually contain none of the active ingredient. The reactions of both groups will be analyzed and compared. Of course neither group is told which is the control group.

Random selection   When the entire population of test subjects has been assembled, the group will be divided into control and test sections by means of a statistical random selection procedure. In this way no claims can be made that subjects in one group were substantially different—sicker, more healthy, older, younger—from subjects in the other.

Evaluation   When the study has been completed, the findings are collected and subjected to statistical analysis. In this way it becomes possible to determine if the results occurred by chance alone or were a consequence of the new item or technique being tested. This step is a critical one in analyzing any new product or test method.

Results   The final step is the publication in a medical journal of the entire study, including both the analysis and conclusion. Before this article can appear in print, it must first be passed through the final test: a written review by experts in the field. Once it has been put through these demanding paces then, and only then, should it be released to the public.

The Fallacy Behind the Anecdote

As you can see, the demands made on medical researchers are rigorous and extremely objective; and well they should be, as the outcome of these tests involves significant matters of health and disease. Indeed, it can be said that any medical procedure that has not been put through this sequence of tests is unproven and should not be commercially available to the general public.

Unfortunately, there are a number of such unproven procedures and clinical practices in use today, several of which have recently achieved a degree of attention—if not respectability—within limited sectors of the medical community. The differences between these controversial practices and those which have become standard among allergists are significant and stem principally from the question of *proof*. What does this mean exactly? As I stated earlier, the scientific method requires that data obtained from group experiments be mathematically analyzed by the latest in statistical methods before it can be certified for use on patients. This is in keeping with the scientific method. On the other hand, physicians who utilize what have been termed controversial procedures rely on quite another system of reporting which, in the opinion of most physicians, falls far short of objectivity. It is the so-called anecdotal method.

Anecdotal? In fact, we have all heard such reports, stories about how at such-and-such a clinic physicians have had a 75 percent recovery rate for cancer, about how Dr. P——— has healed thousands of cases of incurable arthritis with his secret elixirs, and so forth. Technically, an example coming directly from a doctor might read as follows: "In my experience, nine out of ten patients taking drug X have shown definite clinical improvement." This sounds good, but where is the information regarding the use of a control group? Where is the statistical analysis? Where are the reviews and opinions by experts in the field? Where are the other physicians who have used the same methods and derived the same satisfactory results? Usually they are absent. All we have is one doctor's testimony, plus the testimony of a number of patients, all or any of whom may have been cured by suggestion, by the body's natural healing processes, by accident, by the placebo effect, by a half-dozen variables, none of which were actually brought about by the specific procedure itself.

The fact is that a single doctor's experience with a procedure can *never* stand alone as adequate medical testimony. The controversial procedure in question may indeed work, it may indeed cure; but then again, it may only *seem* to work. How can we tell the difference when a handful of practitioners have claimed wonderful results with the method while others simply cannot achieve the same success? If there is only anectodal evidence in support of an otherwise unproven technique, a new patient should think it over very carefully before agreeing to undergo testing or treatment using an undocumented method. I believe, in fact, that more harm has been done to patients on both an emotional and financial level by the false raising of hopes than the possible small good such methods may have contributed through the placebo effect.

Controversial Practices in Allergic Medicine

Cytotoxic Testing

Cytotoxic testing is a procedure that requires the taking of approximately two teaspoonfuls of blood (10 cc) from the patient. In the lab the white blood cells are separated from the red cells and the serum; a portion of the patient's white cell suspension is placed on a slide along with a specific dried food allergen—say, for peanut. A few drops of fluid are added and the slide is observed under a microscope. So far, so good. A positive reaction indicating a "peanut allergy" can then supposedly be determined by what happens to the white blood cells. If they change their usual shape, slow down their normally active motion or disintegrate, an allergic sensitivity to that particular food is said to be proven.

It all sounds great—if only it were true. Today this test is being performed by laboratories and individual physicians in many of the major metropolitan centers around the country. It has been extensively advertised in both professional and lay publications and is frequently reported as being a "state-of-the-art technique" for diagnosing a whole list of supposedly "allergic" symptoms —which is even more ironic, as this particular method has been known and written about for approximately forty years.

Where, in my opinion and in the opinion of other allergists, does cytotoxic testing go wrong? Generally speaking, the test is used to diagnose food allergies and to identify the symptoms that reputedly accompany them. These symptoms include headache, skin rashes, nausea and other responses not necessarily characteristic of allergic reactions, such as heart palpitations and chronic insomnia. Champions of cytotoxic testing go so far as to claim that many apparently unrelated symptoms such as stress, depression and even backaches can all actually be the result of allergic reactions to food. They maintain that cytotoxic testing will determine which of these foods is really to blame.

All this would also be well and good, if it were true. From a number of well-controlled studies the following contrary facts have been made clear:

Results of cytotoxic testing done on the same patient on two separate days produced entirely different clinical results.

Technicians working in different rooms studying the same cytotoxic test slides under the microscope were unable to agree on the results.

Test results were unable to differentiate between foods which caused a clinical allergy in a patient as compared with foods which caused no problems when eaten by the same patient.

In California, a specimen of blood obtained from a cow was sent to a laboratory for evaluation. The report from the laboratory stated that the patient was indeed allergic—to milk!

Finally, in an evaluation of all the existing studies made to date, the American Academy of Allergy and Immunology, an organization composed of recognized specialists in the field of allergic medicine, concluded that cytotoxic testing is "unproven, unreliable and without scientific basis." The Food and Drug Administration in April 1985 stated that cytotoxic testing is "unreliable as a diagnostic test."

Autogenous Urine Immunization

This technique involves the intramuscular injection of a patient's own urine after the urine has been sterilized and filtered under laboratory conditions. If such a bizarre procedure sounds suspect, it is. Fortunately, this method is rarely used today, and indeed, it should never be used. Not only is there absolutely *no* evidence that urine injections are beneficial for allergic conditions (or for any other conditions, for that matter), but using such a technique can make the patient a candidate for a dangerous kidney disease called nephritis. For this reason the American Academy of Allergy and Immunology has issued a warning stating that autogenous urine immunization techniques are potentially dangerous to your health. If you were—or are—considering such a procedure for your child, my only word of advice on the subject is, don't!

Rinkel Method

Those allergists who use the Rinkel technique, which is supposed to determine the safe starting dose as well as the highest maintenance level for an immunotherapy ("allergy shot") treatment program, have not proven their claims.

At first glance, this may sound like a technical argument for doctors only, and to some extent it is. But the question directly affects the patient as well. For any individual the maintenance or top dose that the Rinkel method states is appropriate is far too weak to provide the patient with positive results. If your child is about to begin an immunotherapy program, which usually takes years to complete, you as the parent need to know that the treatment will be effective. Indeed, the American Academy of Allergy and Immunology has analyzed the results of several studies done on the Rinkel method and has come to the conclusion that the maximum dose suggested by this method is far too low to be medically useful. There was no evidence to prove that "this method is an effective guide to determine the optimal therapeutic dose for immunotherapy." It has even been found in at least one well-controlled study that there was no difference between a placebo and the "optimum therapeutic dose" called for by the Rinkel method." This technique, under certain circumstances, recommends a top treatment dose that is so weak that the prospect of it helping the patient would be extremely unlikely.

Provocation and Neutralization Testing

As the name suggests, this method is designed to first provoke allergic symptoms in a patient (provocation) and then, in the second phase of treatment, to neutralize these symptoms and cause them to entirely disappear (neutralization). Those physicians who use this procedure claim that it is effective for both diagnosing and treating allergic conditions.

The first stage, the provocation part, is started either by the subcutaneous injection of the suspected allergen or by placing the extract directly under the child's tongue (sublingual). The allergen is administered in increasing strength until the supposed allergy-caused symptoms make their appearance.

Now for the neutralization stage. Here a "neutralization dose" is given which contains the same material used in the provocation dose but in a much weaker dilution. This part of the procedure can be done either by placing the allergen under the tongue (sublingual neutralization) or by injecting the substance (subcutaneous neutralization). This extract may also be administered by injection or under the tongue, and, according to its champions, it will quickly eliminate all allergic symptoms.

Once again, when this method was studied in a controlled fashion under appropriate laboratory conditions, investigators were unable to document either its ability to diagnose or treat allergic conditions. By the way, this procedure has been recommended and marketed as a very effective way of diagnosing and treating food allergies. Unfortunately, it doesn't work! The American Academy of Allergy and Immunology stated that provocation and neutralization methods are definitely "unproven." They also concluded that "no known immunologic mechanism" could account for any symptoms being neutralized by the highly diluted antigen extracts used in this procedure. The academy recommends that this test be considered an experimental procedure only and nothing more.

A Final Word on Controversial Practices

I realize that it is extremely difficult for the parents of allergic children to read about so-called medical breakthroughs for asthma or so-called state-of-the-art food allergy therapies without being swayed. All I can advise is that before you spend your time, effort and money on one of these promised cures—and before you decide to opt for such methods at the expense of proven therapeutic procedures—you do a bit of investigating on your own.

Where? And how? Start with your local Better Business Bureau. You may be surprised to learn how many dubious and sometimes even fraudulent medical practices advertise in legitimate newspapers, journals and magazines. Also check with local medical societies. Make inquiries concerning the test or procedure in question. Ask the society if they recommend it. Find out if it is an accepted medical practice or if it is still in the evaluation or experimental phase.

Medical schools can help; some even maintain information services designed to answer queries concerning controversial medical practices. Ask whatever questions seem appropriate and important. Does the physician or the laboratory who performs this test have a good reputation? Is he or she properly licensed? Has the method been published and reviewed in legitimate medical journals? Are the claims medically justified? Why? Why not? Has there been any trouble?

Don't be afraid to question the doctor or the laboratory that administers this test, and don't hestitate to walk out if their answers are unsatisfactory. Many of these controversial techniques are expensive, and an increasing number of insurance companies are refusing to honor claims made for procedures that are unproven or experimental. If you are spending your time, effort and money on one of these unproven methods, you will almost certainly be depriving your child of the benefits scientifically documented standard allergy treatment can provide. As P. T. Barnum is reputed to have said: "There's a sucker born every minute." As far as medical matters go, make sure you and your children are not among them.

Allergic Emergencies

One of the most frightening medical experiences for patient, parents and physician is a generalized allergic response, technically known as an anaphylactic reaction. This is a true medical emergency, during which the patient develops intense generalized itching, swelling of virtually any part of the body, especially the face, tongue and throat, along with severe breathing problems. If untreated it can lead to shock, severe respiratory distress and death. Over the past twenty years I have treated children who were in anaphylactic shock; certain cases stand out clearly. One of them, a seven-year-old boy named Larry whom I had known for a half year or so, was brought to my office twenty minutes after being stung by a yellow jacket. Normally a bright penny of a boy, Larry now resembled a grotesque caricature of himself, his face swollen to practically twice its normal size, his skin covered with giant hives that itched uncontrollably, his lungs so congested that each breath had become a labored gasp.

Larry responded dramatically to treatment with Adrenalin, oxygen and antihistamines, and within two or three hours he was on his way home. He had to stay on medication for several days after the episode, and the psychological shock of this life-threatening experience left its mark not only on Larry but on his entire family.

The point is that an anaphylactic reaction is a highly traumatic experience for *everyone,* patient, parents and attending physician alike. The message from Larry's case history that you must never forget is that *immediate medical attention must be given as soon as possible after generalized symptoms appear.*

This point cannot be emphasized too strongly. Anaphylaxis is a very serious condition, even a potentially fatal one, and it must be attended to rapidly or serious consequences will almost certainly occur. Unless you have proper medical training and have the appropriate drugs at home to treat an anaphylactic reaction, get your child to the nearest doctor or hospital *as soon as possible.* You are courting potential disaster if you attempt to manage this situation without medical assistance. In this chapter I will provide you with information on the causes, course and management of acute allergic reactions, focusing specifically on anaphylaxis. You can then use this information to recognize an allergic emergency quickly and act on it.

Recognizing an Allergic Medical Emergency

How frequently do anaphylactic reactions occur? While completely accurate statistics concerning this question are not available, it is possible to review those figures that have been published to get a general idea of how prevalent this problem is.

> Fatal anaphylactic reactions will occur yearly to approximately 4 out of every 10 million people. This means that, statistically, with a population of roughly 240 million people in the United States, around 100 people per year will die of anaphylaxis. The actual number is almost certainly a good deal higher.
>
> The number of *nonfatal* anaphylactic episodes in the United States ranges from 50 to 500 times higher than for fatal anaphylaxis. This means there may be as many as 50,000 cases a year of nonfatal anaphylactic shock.
>
> Depending on which textbook or article you read, the number of fatalities attributed to anaphylactic reactions *from penicillin alone* ranges from 500 to 1000 deaths per year.
>
> Fatal reactions resulting from X-ray contrast media is estimated in one study to be as high as 500 per year.

From these few figures it is clear that anaphylaxis is a significant problem. Let me stress again, however, that while severe, it can ordinarily be controlled if prompt appropriate medical treatment is received. We may, in fact, assume that many of these reported fatalities occurred because of the victim's inability to gain medical help quickly or because he failed to recognize the seriousness of his symptoms until it was too late.

What determines whether a particular anaphylactic reaction will be serious or moderate? Two factors: the degree of sensitivity which the person has to the specific allergen, and the route by which the allergen enters the body. The first rule speaks for itself. The second, in practical terms, means that a child who is allergic to penicillin runs a much greater risk of reaction if the penicillin is injected rather than taken by mouth, and that a substance taken intravenously is more likely to produce a rapid and violent reaction than one received orally.

The areas most commonly involved during a generalized allergic reaction include the respiratory tract, the skin, the gastrointestinal tract and the cardiovascular system. The symptoms associated with each of these organ systems are as follows:

Respiratory Tract

Runny nose with profuse, clear, watery discharge.

A sensation of swelling in the throat, as though the throat were closing up.

A hoarse voice.

A tight feeling in the chest and a progressive inability to draw air into the lungs.

A tight cough associated with shortness of breath and wheezing.

If the reaction continues without appropriate treatment, respiratory arrest can occur.

The Skin

While skin symptoms tend to be generalized, they often begin at the injection site in the form of a red, itchy rash.

Hives. These may be small, individual lesions, or they may flow together to cover entire sections of the body.

Distortion and swelling of the facial features due to angioedema.

Severe generalized itching with a red rash over most of the body.

Gastrointestinal Tract

Severe abdominal pain and cramping caused by swelling in the intestinal tract.

Nausea.

Vomiting.

Explosive diarrhea (which is sometimes bloody).

Cardiovascular Systems

A sudden drop in blood pressure.

Irregular heartbeat.

Cardiac arrest (during the most severe episodes).

Other Symptoms

An indefinable sense of impending disaster, a strange feeling that something terrible is about to take place. This sensation may come over the patient even if the symptoms are not yet apparent.

Convulsions.

Death due to anaphylaxis in children is relatively rare; most fatalities of this kind take place among the adult population. When death does occur to youngsters, it is usually due to severe swelling of the throat (laryngeal edema), which makes it impossible to breathe. It should be mentioned, too, that a patient can have a milder, nonfatal form of anaphylactic reaction. In fact, when generalized reactions do take place, you can rest assured that if proper steps are taken, the vast majority of cases will be controlled without serious consequences.

Finally, a note on the difference between anaphylaxis and anaphylactoid reactions. Briefly, while the symptoms of an anaphylactoid reaction and those of an anaphylactic reaction are practically the same, the causes are different. Anaphylactoid reactions are not IgE antibody–mediated responses—that is, they do not involve an antigen-antibody reaction. From a clinical point of view there is no way to tell the difference between these two reactions. Treatment is the same for both situations, and the response to medication is similar.

How to Deal with an Allergic Emergency

Two important questions about allergic emergencies:

> What can I do if I suspect that a family member is having an anaphylactic reaction?
> What should the doctor do for a person having an anaphylactic reaction?

First question first: As a parent, probably the best thing you can do for your child, besides learning to recognize symptoms in advance, is to *not panic.* There is nothing more frightening for a youngster than the awareness that his parents are uncertain how to respond to his problem. If *you* can't help me, she thinks to herself, who can? Thus, even if you are not entirely sure of how to handle this difficult situation, *act as if you did,* at least until medical help has arrived. Most of all, stay clear-headed, deliberate and sympathetic. Even if you are not calm, try to act that way. Your calmness will help your child.

As soon as you suspect that your child is having an anaphylactic reaction, here's what you must do:

> Give an antihistamine. Chances are there will be one somewhere in the medicine cabinet, especially if your child has a history of allergy.

> Observe your child for any swallowing difficulties (swelling of the throat or a change in voice quality) or problems in breathing such as shortness of breath or wheezing.

> If there is any evidence of respiratory distress or swallowing difficulty, get your child to a doctor's office or an emergency room, and do it *immediately.* This situation is dangerous—this is a true medical emergency!

> If there are no breathing or swallowing problems, and if a trip to a medical facility is not required, stay in touch with your doctor for additional directions.

What if your child's symptoms become so severe that you must go to the hospital? What can you expect once you arrive? More or less the following:

A doctor will quickly examine and evaluate your child to determine the severity of the symptoms.

Treatment will be started. In most cases the drug epinephrine (Adrenalin) will be used first. The dose will be determined by the patient's weight.

A second injection of epinephrine will usually be administered within twenty to thirty minutes after the first. (A patient can be given up to three injections of epinephrine at twenty- to thirty-minute intervals.) An antihistamine may also be given orally or by injection.

Most patients will respond dramatically to the epinephrine. If there is any evidence of cyanosis caused by insufficient oxygen reaching the bloodstream, oxygen may also be administered. This will be given either by a face mask or by nasal prongs fitted directly into the nose.

For the majority of patients, combined treatment with epinephrine, antihistamines and oxygen will bring the anaphylactic reaction under control. Patients will continue to take antihistamines until all symptoms have disappeared; this is usually for one to three days.

If outpatient treatment is not successful in controlling the symptoms your child may have to be admitted to the hospital for more intensive therapy. Such treatment usually entails the administration of intravenous medications to raise blood pressure and control wheezing. Cortisone preparations will also be given to decrease both the severity and the duration of symptoms. If a period of hospitalization is necessary, it will rarely exceed two or three days. Most commonly an overnight admission is all that is required.

What Causes Anaphylaxis?

Throughout this book I have referred to the types of generalized reactions which may result from various allergic conditions. For specifics on the causes and etiology of these difficulties, I refer you to the various chapters on asthma, food allergy, skin conditions, rhinitis, insect stings and so on. To briefly review the subject, the following list of biological and chemical substances, though certainly not all-inclusive, represents a majority of the major offenders:

insect venom (see the chapter on insect stings)
penicillin (see the chapter on adverse drug reactions)
allergy extract treatment materials (see the chapter on adverse drug reactions)
vaccines made from horse serum (see the chapter on adverse drug reactions)
X-ray contrast media (see the chapter on adverse drug reactions)

local anesthetics such as Procaine and Lidocaine (see the chapter on adverse drug reactions)

foods such as milk, eggs, shellfish, nuts, chocolate and fish (see the chapter on food allergies)

aspirin (see the chapter on adverse drug reactions)

chemicals added to foods such as dyes, colorings, stabilizers, emulsifiers and preservatives (see the chapters on adverse drug reactions and food allergies)

For an allergic individual, any of these substances can become the trigger for an anaphylactic reaction. Once someone in your family has had such a response, it is strongly recommended that he wear a tag or necklace identifying the allergy; information on Medic Alert bracelets can be found at most pharmacies. Finally—and repeating what has already been said several times—in the event of an anaphylactic reaction, the most important things you or anyone else can do for the victim are the following:

Stay calm.
Give an antihistamine.
Call the doctor.
If the symptoms become progressively worse, take the patient immediately to the nearest medical facility.

This is the key to success in treating any allergic emergency—quick recognition followed by rapid response and prompt medical attention.

Appendix

Asthma Chronic Care Centers

A small percentage of children with asthma have symptoms which are so severe that they can only be adequately treated in a residential asthma treatment center. This appendix contains the names and addresses of these centers.

United States

California
Stanford Children's Convalescent
    Hospital
Allergy Service
520 Willow Road
Palo Alto, CA 94304
(415) 327-4800

Colorado
National Asthma Center, combined
    with National Jewish Hospital
1999 Julian Street
Denver, CO 80204
(303) 458-1999

District of Columbia
Hospital for Sick Children
1731 Bunker Hill Road NE
Washington, DC 20017
(202) 832-4400

Illinois
La Rabida Children's Hospital and
    Research Center
65th Street at Lake Michigan
Chicago, IL 60649
(312) 363-6700

Maryland
Mount Washington Pediatric
    Hospital
1708 West Rogers Avenue
Baltimore, MD 21209
(301) 578-8600

Massachusetts
Lakeville Hospital Asthma
    Rehabilitation Unit
Main Street
Lakeville, MA 02346
(617) 947-1231

Michigan
Mary Free Bed Hospital and
    Rehabilitation Center
235 Wealthy Street SE
Grand Rapids, MI 49503
(616) 774-6774

New Jersey
Betty Bacharach Rehabilitation
    Center
4100 Atlantic Avenue
Pomona, NJ 08240
(609) 652-7000

Children's Seashore House
Jim Leeds Road
Atlantic City, NJ 08401
(609) 345-5191

New York
St. Mary's Hospital for Children
29-01 216th Street
Bayside, NY 11360
(718) 990-8870

New York Infirmary
321 East 15th Street
New York, NY 10003
(212) 228-8000

Blythedale Children's Hospital
Bradhurst Avenue
Valhalla, NY 10595
(914) 592-7555

Asthmatic Children's Foundation
Spring Valley Road
Ossining, New York 10562
(914) 762-2110

Ohio
Convalescent Hospital for Children
    Asthmatic Unit at Children's
    Hospital
Elland and Bethesda Avenues
Cincinnati, OH 45229
(513) 559-4200

Health Hill Hospital for Children
2801 East Boulevard
Cleveland, OH 44104
(216) 721-5400

Oklahoma
Children's Convalescent Center
P.O. Box 888
6800 Northwest 39th Expressway
Bethany, OK 73008
(405) 789-6711

Pennsylvania
Children's Heart Hospital
Conshohocken Road
Philadelphia, PA 19131
(215) 877-7708

Canada

Ontario Crippled Children's Centre
350 Rumsey Road
Toronto, Ontario
(416) 425-6220

Queen Alexandra Hospital
2400 Arbutus Road

Vancouver, British Columbia
V8N 1V7
(604) 477-1826

Sunny Hill Hospital for Children
3644 Slocan Street
Vancouver, British Columbia
(604) 434-1331

Summer Camps for Asthmatic Children

It is my personal opinion that the vast majority of children who have asthma can spend their summer vacation at a regular camp. It is not necessary for most asthmatic youngsters to go to a camp which specializes in caring for children who have this condition. There is only a small percentage of children whose asthma is so severe that it would be in their best interests to attend a summer camp which has both the staff and medical facilities to adequately care for them.

The following list will provide you with the names and locations of camps which have a special interest in seeing that asthmatic children enjoy the wonderful experiences available at a summer camp.

As in choosing any summer camp, I recommend that you meet with the camp director and if possible visit the camp before deciding that "this is the right place" for your child.

Summer Camps

California
Allergy Foundation of Northern
    California
(Santa Cruz Mountains)
141 Camino Alto
Mill Valley, CA 94941

Camp Wheez
277 West Hedding Street
San Jose, CA 95110

Scamp Camp
(Running Springs, CA)
3861 Front Street
San Diego, CA 92103

Sunair Children's Camp
1670 Beverly Boulevard
Los Angeles, CA 90026

Colorado
Champ Camp
(Estes Park, CO)
1600 Race Street
Denver, CO 80206

Florida
Camp Sunshine Station
(Melrose, FL)
Florida Lung Association
P.O. Box 8127

Jacksonville, FL 32211

Illinois
Camp Tapawango
(Peoria, IL)
1 Christmas Seal Drive
Springfield, IL 62703

Camp Superkids
(Iowa)
1321 Walnut Street
Des Moines, IL 50309

Kentucky
Camp Weasel
University of Kentucky Medical
    Center
Lexington, KY 40506

Missouri
Camp Sun Deer
(Battle Creek, MI)
American Lung Association of
    Southeastern Michigan
28 West Adams Street
Detroit, MI 48226

Minnesota
Wilderness Camp
(Northern Minnesota)
American Lung Association of
    Hennepin County

1829 Portland Avenue
Minneapolis, MN 55404

North Dakota
Camp Superkids, Triangle and
    Camp Sakawea
(Garrison, ND)
212 North 2nd Street
Bismarck, ND 58501

Nebraska
Camp Superkids
(Nebraska)
7363 Pacific Street
Suite 212
Omaha, NE 68114

New Hampshire
YMCA Camp Foss
(Barnstead, NH)
456 Beech Street
Manchester, NH 03105

New Mexico
Camp Superkids
(Sante Fe, NM)
216 Truman Avenue, N.E.
Albuquerque, NM 87108

New York
Camp Massawixie
(Adirondack Mountains)
Boy Scout Council of Monroe
    County
474 East Avenue
Rochester, NY 14607

Camp Superkids
23 South Street
Utica, NY 13501

Oklahoma
Camp Superstuff
(Sapula, OK)
5553 South Peoria
Tulsa, OK 74105

Oregon
Camp Christmas Seal
Oregon Lung Association
1020 S.W. Taylor
Suite 830
Portland, OR 97205

Virginia
Camp Holiday Trails
P.O. Box 5806
Charlottesville, VA 22903

Allergy Clinics

This is a representative listing of the allergy clinics found at university medical training centers and larger hospitals throughout the country. If you do not find a listing for your city or state, additional information regarding allergy treatment centers can be obtained by contacting your local medical society.

Arkansas
University of Arkansas Medical
    Center
4301 West Markham Street
Little Rock, AR 72201
(501) 661-5000

California
Scripps Clinic and Research
    Foundation
476 Prospect Street
La Jolla, CA 92037
(619) 455-9100

Los Angeles–USC Medical Center
1200 North State Street
Los Angeles, CA 90033
(213) 226-6503

UCLA Hospital
10833 Le Conte Avenue
Los Angeles, CA 90024
(213) 825-6481

University of California-Irvine
	Medical Center
101 City Drive South
Orange, CA 92668
(714) 634-6011

Children's Hospital at Stanford
520 Willow Road
Palo Alto, CA 94304
(415) 327-4800

University Hospital
University of California Medical
	Center
225 West Dickinson Street
San Diego, CA 92103
(619) 294-6222

Kaiser Foundation Hospital
2200 O'Farrell
San Francisco, CA 94115
(415) 929-4000

University of California Hospitals
	and Clinics
513 Parnassus Avenue
San Francisco, CA 94143
(415) 666-9000

Stanford University Medical Center
300 Pasteur Drive
Stanford, CA 94305
(415) 497-2300

Harbor General Hospital
1000 West Carson Street
Torrance, CA 90509
(213) 533-2104

Colorado
Fitzsimons Army Medical Center
Peoria and Colfax Streets
Denver, CO 80240
(303) 361-8241

National Asthma Center
1999 Julian Street
Denver, CO 80204
(303) 458-1999

National Jewish Hospital
3800 East Colfax Avenue
Denver, CO 80206
(303) 388-4461

University of Colorado Medical
	Center
4200 East Ninth Avenue
Denver, CO 80262
(303) 394-7601

Connecticut
Yale–New Haven Medical Center
333 Cedar Street
New Haven, CT 06510
(203) 436-8060

District of Columbia
Children's Hospital National
	Medical Center
111 Michigan Avenue
Washington, DC 20010
(202) 745-5000

Georgetown University Hospital
3800 Reservoir Road, NW
Washington, DC 20007
(202) 625-7001

Howard University Hospital
2041 Georgia Avenue, NW
Washington, DC 20060
(202) 745-1596

Florida
William A. Shands Teaching
    Hospital and Clinics
University of Florida
Gainesville, FL 32610
(904) 392-3771

Illinois
Children's Memorial Hospital
2300 Children's Plaza
Chicago, IL 60614
(312) 880-4000

Institute of Allergy and Clinical
    Immunology
Grant Hospital of Chicago
550 West Webster Avenue
Chicago, IL 60614
(312) 883-2000

Michael Reese Hospital and
    Medical Center
508 East 29th Street
Chicago, IL 60616
(312) 791-2000

Northwestern University Memorial
    Hospital
Superior Street and Fairbanks
    Court
Chicago, IL 60611
(312) 649-8624

Rush-Presbyterian-St. Luke's
    Medical Center
1753 West Congress Parkway
Chicago, IL 60612
(312) 942-5000

University of Illinois Hospital
1919 West Taylor Street
Chicago, IL 60612
(312) 996-7000

Iowa
University of Iowa Hospitals and
    Clinics
650 Newton Road
Iowa City, IA 52242
(391) 356-1616

Kansas
University of Kansas College of
    Health Sciences and Bell
    Memorial Hospital
39th Street and Rainbow Boulevard
Kansas City, KS 66103
(913) 588-6008

Louisiana
Tulane University School of
    Medicine
Allergy Clinic
1430 Tulane Avenue
New Orleans, LA 70112
(504) 588-5578

Maryland
Good Samaritan Hospital
5601 Loch Raven Boulevard
Baltimore, MD 21239
(301) 323-2200

Johns Hopkins Hospital
601 North Broadway
Baltimore, MD 21205
(301) 955-5000

Massachusetts
Children's Hospital Medical Center
300 Longwood Avenue
Boston, MA 02115
(617) 734-6000

Massachusetts General Hospital
  Clinical Immunology and
  Allergy Unit
Fruit Street
Boston, MA 02114
(617) 726-2000

Robert B. Brigham Hospital
125 Parker Hill Avenue
Boston, MA 02120
(617) 732-5055

Michigan
University Hospital
1405 East Ann Street
Ann Arbor, MI 48109
(313) 764-3184

Henry Ford Hospital
2799 West Grand Boulevard
Detroit, MI 48202
(313) 876-2600

Minnesota
University of Minnesota Hospitals
  and Clinics
516 Delaware Street
Minneapolis, MN 55455
(612) 373-8484

Mayo Clinic and Foundation
200 First Street SW
Rochester, MN 55901
(507) 284-2511

Missouri
Children's Mercy Hospital
24th Street and Gillham Road
Kansas City, MO 64108
(816) 234-3000

Barnes Hospital–Washington
  University Medical School
Barnes Hospital Plaza

St. Louis, MO 63110
(314) 454-2000

St. Louis University Medical Center
1402 South Grand Boulevard
St. Louis, MO 63104
(314) 664-9800

Nebraska
St. Joseph Hospital
(formerly Creighton Hospital)
601 North 30th Street
Omaha, NE 68131
(402) 449-4001

New York
Interfaith Medical Center
555 Prospect Plaza
Brooklyn, NY 11238
(212) 240-1761

Children's Hospital of Buffalo
219 Bryant Street
Buffalo, NY 14222
(716) 878-7000

Nassau County Medical Center
2201 Hempstead Turnpike
East Meadow, NY 11554
(516) 542-0123

R. A. Cooke Institute of Allergy—
  Roosevelt Hospital
428 West 59th Street
New York, NY 10028
(212) 554-7000

Cornell Medical School—New York
  Hospital
510 East 70th Street
New York, NY 10021
(212) 472-5900

Columbia-Presbyterian Medical
    Center
622 West 168th Street
New York, NY 10032
(212) 305-2300

New York University Medical
    Center
552 First Avenue
New York, NY 10016
(212) 340-5241

Strong Memorial Hospital of the
    University of Rochester
601 Elmwood Avenue
Rochester, NY 14642
(716) 275-2121

North Carolina
Duke University Medical Center
Durham, NC 27710
(919) 684-8111

Ohio
Children's Hospital Medical Center
Elland and Bethesda Avenues
Cincinnati, OH 45229
(513) 559-4200

Cleveland Clinic Foundation
9500 Euclid Avenue
Cleveland, OH 44106
(216) 444-5780

Ohio State University Hospitals
456 Clinic Drive
Columbus, OH 43210
(614) 422-4851

Pennsylvania
Children's Hospital of Philadelphia
34th Street and Civic Center
    Boulevard
Philadelphia, PA 19104
(215) 596-9100

Hahnemann Medical College and
    Hospital
Feinstein Building
216 North Broad Street
Philadelphia, PA 19102
(215) 448-7000

Hospital of University of
    Pennsylvania
34th and Spruce Streets
Philadelphia, PA 19104
(215) 662-4000

Thomas Jefferson University
    Hospital
11th and Walnut Streets
Philadelphia, PA 19107
(215) 928-6000

Children's Hospital of Pittsburgh
125 De Soto Street
Pittsburgh, PA 15213
(412) 647-2345

Rhode Island
Rhode Island Hospital
593 Eddy Street
Providence, RI 02902
(401) 277-4000

Texas
University of Texas Health Sciences
    Center
7703 Floyd Curl Drive
San Antonio, TX 78284
(512) 691-6011

University of Texas Medical Branch
    Hospitals
8th and Mechanic Streets
Galveston, TX 77550
(713) 765-1011

Texas Children's Hospital—Baylor
  College of Medicine
6621 Fannin
Houston, TX 77030
(713) 791-4219

Virginia
University of Virginia Hospitals
Private Clinic Building
Hospital Drive
Charlottesville, VA 22908
(804) 924-0211

Medical College of Virginia
  Hospitals
12th and Marshall Streets
Richmond, VA 23298
(804) 786-9000

Washington
University Hospital
1959 Northeast Pacific Street
Seattle, WA 98195
(206) 543-3300

Wisconsin
University of Wisconsin Hospital
  and Clinics
600 Highland Avenue
Madison, WI 53702
(608) 263-8000

Milwaukee County Medical
  Complex
8700 West Wisconsin Avenue
Milwaukee, WI 53226
(414) 257-5915

Asthma and Allergy Foundation of America Chapters and Chapter Presidents

California
Los Angeles Chapter, AAFA
Scott McCreary
Executive Director
Suite 1005
5410 Wilshire Blvd.
Los Angeles, CA 90036
(213) 937-7859
  Marj Malloy
  President
  7843 Woodrow Wilson Dr.
  Los Angeles, CA 90046
  (213) 654-2077

Orange County Chapter
  Ken Weir
  President
  2709 South El Camino Real
  San Clemente, CA 92672

(714) 496-2749 (h)
(714) 492-7240 (w)

Redwood Empire Chapter
c/o Dr. Roger Barron
2461 Summerfield Road
Santa Rosa, CA 95405
(707) 523-4426
(707) 525-0211
  Treasurer's Mail
  Jane Rinehart
  2461 Summerfield Road
  Santa Rosa, CA 95405

District of Columbia
Metropolitan Washington Chapter
c/o Liz Sheuble
2921 DuBarry Lane
Brookeville, MD 20833
(301) 774-7325

Florida
South Florida Chapter
20900 Biscayne Road
Suite 544
Miami, FL 33180
  Mrs. Karen Froman
  President
  Send large parcels or
  UPS to:
  3901 N. 49th Avenue
  Hollywood, FL 33021
  (305) 931-2299
  (305) 962-6250

Illinois
Greater Chicago Chapter
Suite 909
111 North Wabash
Chicago, IL 60602
  Mailing Address:
  Patricia Koutouzos
  President
  113 Wolpers Road
  Park Forest, IL 60466
  (312) 747-0533

Maryland
Maryland Chapter
Beverly Caporossi
Executive Secretary
5601 Loch Raven Blvd.
Baltimore, MD 21239
(301) 532-4135
Phillip S. Norman, M.D.
President

Massachusetts
New England Chapter
221 Longwood Avenue
Boston, MA 02115
(617) 734-4290
  Cynthia Daley
  President

Send packages or certified mail to:
12 Sheffield West
Winchester, MA 01890
(617) 729-4846

Missouri
St. Louis Chapter
#5 Southmoor
Clayton, MO 63105
(314) 965-5153
  Rae Porter
  President
  (314) 727-0573 (home)
(All mail for Rae is to be mailed to
  her home)
UPS or Special Delivery should be
  mailed to Shirley O'Connor's
  address:
130 Glen Cove
Chesterfield, MO 63017

"Show Me" Chapter
Gail Tucker
Executive Director
339 Jones
Warrensburg, MO 64093
(816) 747-6930
  Maurine Achauer, Ph.D.
  President
  P.O. Box 181
  Warrensburg, MO 64093

Pennsylvania
Southeastern Pennsylvania Chapter
P.O. Box 429
Plymouth Meeting, PA 19462
(215) 825-0852
All UPS or Special Delivery should
  be mailed to:
  Edward K. Tryon
  President
  528 Brookside Avenue
  St. Davids, PA 19087
  (215) 293-1625 (h)
  (215) 557-1536 (w)

Tennessee
East Tennessee Chapter
P.O. Box 11289
Knoxville, TN 37919
(619) 584-AAFA
  Alicia Hardin
  President
  10033 Westland Drive
  Concord, TN 37919
  (615) 966-2973

Provisional Chapters

Florida
Central Florida Chapter
Roth Brothers
P.O. Box 15676
Tampa, FL 33684
(813) 961-8823
(813) 962-2938
  Sandy Roth
  President
  8509 Sun State Street
  Tampa, FL 33684
  (813) 933-1446 (h)
  (813) 885-5811 (w)
  (305) 485-3184 (h)
  (305) 566-2984 (w)

Michigan
Michigan Chapter
P.O. Box 22026
Lansing, MI 48909
  Don Massnick
  President
  112 Hart Street
  Essexville, MI 48732
  (517) 894-2472

Minnesota
c/o Marilee Miller
President
Gustaves Adolphus College
Department of Nursing

507 Capitol Blvd.
St. Paul, MN 55103
(612) 221-2293 (w)
  c/o Marlene Grandy
  102 East Center Street
  Rochester, MN 55904
  (507) 367-4928 (h)
  (507) 282-8659

Missouri
Greater Kansas City Chapter
7905 East 134th Terrace
Grandview, MO 64030
(816) 763-3319
  Noel Albert
  President

Nebraska
Missouri Valley Chapter
P.O. Box 14931
Omaha, NE 68124
(402) 333-9121
  Steven J. Riekes
  c/o Richards, Riekes,
  Brown & Zabin, P.C.
  300 Overland-Wolf Center
  6910 Pacific Street
  Omaha, NE 68106
  (402) 558-1112

North Carolina
North Carolina Chapter
1903 St. Mary's Street
Raleigh, NC 27608
  Bobbie Musselwhite
  President
  (919) 821-2484

Ohio
Greater Cincinnati Chapter
Richard Remmy
Executive Director
Deaconess Hospital
311 Straight Street

Cincinnati, OH 45219
(513) 559-2618 or 2619
  Don E. Fowls
  President
  5090 Elmcrest Lane
  Cincinnati, OH 45242
  (513) 984-1513

Texas
El Paso Area Chapter
9455 Viscount #407
El Paso, TX 79925
(915) 598-5250
  Frances Thurman
  President
  5209 Spruce Creek Lane
  El Paso, TX 79932
  (915) 584-4946

A Breathing Exercise for Children with Asthma

Belly Breathing

Children should do the belly-breathing exercise (Figure 10) sitting down. Stand behind your child and put your hand on his shoulders.

Massage

Gently massage your child's shoulders, chest, and back. Rub gently in circular motions for several minutes until the child expresses relief or visibly relaxes. The purpose of massage is to have parents and children work together to help each other relax.

Productive Cough

Give your child a tissue. Then ask your child to take a deep breath to open the lungs and airways. Second, have her cough strongly to bring up mucus from deep inside the lungs. Third, remove the mucus with a tissue.

This works well early when wheezing isn't severe. Don't do coughing in the middle of a serious attack: do it early. The child can even do this at school if she finds a private place. Encourage your child and make sure she takes a deep breath, then a big cough. Encourage your child to cough up mucus, not just saliva.

Parents and children can work together to manage an attack at home by doing belly breathing, massage, and productive cough. Belly breathing can help the child relax during an asthma attack or as he takes a breather during exercise. Massage can be used as an alternative form of relaxation if the belly breathing is not working well for the child. The massage can be done in association with productive cough. The sequence of these relaxation exercises is dependent on the personal preference of the child, based on past experience.

Sit up straight in a chair.

Place both hands on your belly.

Breathe in slowly through your nose. As you take the air in, feel your belly blow up like a balloon. Keep your chest still.

Blow the air slowly out of your mouth through puckered lips. Feel your belly get small.

Repeat this exercise slowly ten times or until you get your breath back.

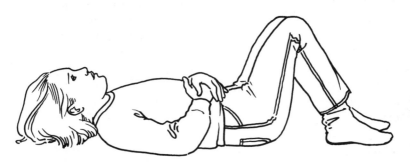

Belly breathing exercise

SOURCE: C.H. Feldman and N.M. Clark, *Open Airways/Respiro Abierto: Asthma Self-Management Program,* National Heart, Lung, and Blood Institute, NIH Publication No. 84-2365.

SOURCE: *National Heart, Lung & Blood Institute*

Food Families

An allergy to one member of a specific food family may mean sensitivity exists to the other foods in the family. Certain families are more likely to have this characteristic, such as the pea and citrus families.

Food	*Other Food Family Members*
Apple	Apple, pear, quince
Aster	Artichoke, chicory, dandelíon, endive, escarole, lettuce, sunflower seeds, tarragon
Banana	Banana, plantain
Beet	Beet, spinach
Beech	Beechnut, chestnut
Buckwheat	Buckwheat, rhubarb, sorrel
Cashew	Cashew nuts, mango, pistachio nuts
Chocolate	Chocolate, cocoa, cola
Citrus	Citron, grapefruit, kumquat, lemon, lime, tangerine
Ginger	Cardamom, ginger, turmeric
Goosefoot	Beet, beet sugar, spinach, swiss chard *See* Beet

Grains	Barley, cane, corn, millet, oats, rice, rye, sorghum, wheat, wild rice
Laurel	Avocado, bay leaves, cinnamon, sassafras
Lily	Asparagus, chives, garlic, leeks, onion, sarsaparilla
Mallow	Cottonseed, okra
Melon (Gourd)	Cantaloupe, casaba melon, cucumber, honeydew melon, persian melon, pumpkin, squash, watermelon
Mint	Basil, horehound, mint, peppermint, rosemary, sage, spearmint
Morning glory	Sweet potato, yam
Mulberry	Blueberry, currants, gooseberry, mulberry
Mustard	Broccoli, Brussels sprouts, cabbage, cauliflower, collards, horseradish, kale, mustard, radish, rutabaga, turnip, watercress
Myrtle	Allspice, guava
Palm	Coconut, date
Parsley	Anise, caraway seed, carrot, celery, celery seed, coriander, cumin, dill, fennel, parsley, parsnip
Pea (Legume or Clover)	Acacia, black-eyed peas, licorice, lima beans, navy beans, peanuts, peas, pinto beans, string beans, tragacanth
Plum	Almond, apricot, cherry, nectarine, peach, plum
Potato	Bell peppers, cayenne peppers, chili peppers, eggplant, paprika, potato, tomato
Rose	Blackberry, boysenberry, loganberry, raspberry, strawberry
Walnut	Butternut, hickory nut, pecan, walnut
Bird	Chicken, duck, goose, pheasant, guinea hen, quail, squab, turkey; the eggs of these birds
Crustaceans	Crabs, crayfish, lobster, shrimp, squid

Fish	(Includes both fresh- and saltwater fish) Bass, catfish, flounder, halibut, perch, pike, salmon, sardine, trout, tuna, whitefish
Mammal	Cow, goat, horse, pig, sheep, and their meat, milk, or by-products
Mollusk	Abalone, clam, mussel, oyster, scallops
Reptile	Rattlesnake, turtle

Sulfite-Containing Substances

Although many manufacturers are removing sulfites from their products, it is very important that all ingredient labels be carefully inspected before purchase. The SULFITEST™ test strips, which that can detect the presence of sulfites in food, are now available. They can be purchased from Center Laboratories, 35 Channel Drive, Port Washington, New York 11050.

Drugs
dexamethasone (Decadron)
epinephrine (Adrenalin)
isoproterenol (Isuprel)
isoetharine solution (Bronkosol)
metaproterenol solution (Alupent, Metaprel)
lidocaine with epinephrine (Xylocaine with epinephrine)

Foods

Fresh Fruits and Vegetables (Those Served in Restaurants)
Avocado dip (guacamole)
Fruit (cut, sliced)
Potatoes (cut)
Salad ingredients (lettuce, coleslaw, tomatoes, carrots, peppers, mush-
    rooms, etc.)

Fish and Shellfish
Dried fish
Fresh shellfish, especially shrimp
Frozen, canned, or dried shellfish (clams, crab, lobster, oyster, scallops,
    shrimp)

Prepared Foods
Canned mushrooms
Dry mix salad dressing

Sauces and gravies
Soups (canned or dried)
Fruits and vegetables (frozen, canned, or dried)
Sauerkraut
Pickles
French fries
Potato chips

Miscellaneous Food Products
Gelatin
Wine vinegar
Misc. baked products (e.g. frozen doughs, corn meal)

Drinks
Beer
Cider
Fruit juices
Wine, foreign and domestic
Juice drinks
Cordials

Sources of Salicylates

Drugs
Alka-Seltzer
Anacin
Anahist
APC (aspirin, phenacetin, caffeine)
Ascriptin tablets
Aspergum
Aspirin
Bayer Children's Cold Tablets
Bromo-Quinine
Bromo-Seltzer
Bufferin
Cama Inlay-Tabs
Congespirin
Coricidin (all forms)
Darvon Compound
Dristan
Ecotrin
Empirin Compound
Equagesic
Excedrin

Fiorinal
4-Way Cold Tablets
Inhiston
Liquiprin
Measurin
Midol
Momentum
Norgesic
Panalgesic
Pepto-Bismol
Percodan tablets
Persistin
Quiet World Analgesic/Sleeping
    Aid
Robaxisal
Sal-Sayne
Stanback
Stanback Analgesic Powders
Teracin
Triaminicin
Trigesic

Vanquish
Viro-Med tablets

Flavorings
Oil of Wintergreen
Vanilla
Antiseptics
Beverages
Candies
Cosmetics
Gum
Lozenges
Mouthwash
Perfumes
Toothpaste

Foods
Almonds
Apples
Apricots
Birch beer
Blackberries
Cherries
Currants
Gooseberries
Grapes
Nectarines
Oranges
Pears
Quinces
Peaches
Plums

Raspberries
Strawberries
Teaberry tea
Wine

Suntan Lotions
Acetyl salicylic acid
Aluminum acetyl salicylate
Ammonium salicylate
Arthropan
Calcium acetyl salicylate
Choline salicylate
Ethyl salicylate
Lithium salicylate
Methyl salicylate
Para-aminosalicylic acid
Phenyl salicylate
Procaine salicylate
Sal ethyl carbonate
Salicylamide
Salicylsalicylic acid
Santyl
Sodium salicylate
Strontium salicylate

Miscellaneous
Methylene disalicylic acid, in
    lubricating oils
Salicylanilide, in anti-mildew agents
Soap in green; wintergreen
    fragrance
Sulfosalicylic acid

Substances Containing Tartrazine

Many manufacturers are removing tartrazine (FD&C Yellow Dye No. 5) from their products, but it is still essential to read all content labels.

This is a partial listing and should serve only as a general guideline. If you have a question as to the contents of a particular product, consult your doctor or the manufacturer.

Cake Mixes
Duncan Hines, some varieties
Pillsbury

Candy
Brach's candy corn
Butterscotch
Chocolate chips
Colored marshmallows

Desserts
Canned, ready-to-eat puddings
Commercial cake frostings
Commercially baked pies
Ice creams and sherbets, some brands
Jell-O brand gelatin
Jell-O brand instant pudding and pie filling
Royal brand gelatin

Drinks
Awake
Gatorade, lime flavor
Imitation lemonade mixes
Tang

Food Allergy

Health food stores in your community or specialty sections in your local supermarket are excellent sources for specialized food products. The companies listed in the "Sources for Specific Diet Information" (page 272) are very helpful if you cannot find certain food items in your area.

A publication entitled "Allergy Products Directory" has extensive listings of specific food products and their sources. It can be purchased from
Prologue Publications
Post Office Box 640
Menlo Park, California 94026

You can also find many diet and food books in your local library that will provide you with a more extensive and varied menu for dealing with your allergic child. Your local librarian can serve as an excellent resource for you in this area.

In some instances you may have to seek the advice and guidance of a dietitian or nutritionist. Be certain that the person you choose has the proper credentials. A referral from your physician is an excellent recommendation.

Of course your allergist will discuss any plans for dietary manipulation with you and make general recommendations regarding menu planning.

Food Allergy Elimination Diets

The choice of a specific elimination diet will depend on which food is suspected of causing the symptoms. As a general rule, a discussion with your child's doctor is recommended before making any major or prolonged diet changes. The elimination diets may be used to determine which food is a possible cause of symptoms. The most common sensitizing foods in order of frequency are egg, milk, seafood, nuts, seeds, chocolate, orange and tomato.

Two diets are listed. These contain entirely different foods with the exception of sugar, salt and gelatin. Common allergens are excluded with the exception of milk on Diet Two. The choice of diet depends on the history and skin tests. The diet you choose will depend on the foods you suspect. Choose the diet that has no foods which you suspect cause allergic symptoms in your child. If there is any food on the diet which you know disagrees with your child, omit it. The diet should be maintained rigidly for two weeks, unless symptoms are aggravated. If this occurs, or if there is no improvement, the other diet may be tried.

When improvement occurs, new foods are added at three-day intervals. Symptoms appearing on the addition of a food to the basic diet are the most significant evidence of food allergy. Such evidence should be checked by reintroducing the suspect food after at least a week's abstinence.

These diets are nutritionally inadequate and should not be maintained without change for longer than two weeks. Vitamins, minerals and drugs should not be taken without asking your doctor.

On Diet One, where milk is not allowed, meat should be given twice a day to insure adequate protein. Calcium may be added. Foods containing preservatives should be avoided.

Wheat-Free Diet

Omit these foods.

Beverages

Malted milk, Postum, coffee substitutes, beer, ale

Bread

All breads including rye, unless 100 percent rye, oatmeal, nut breads, hot breads, French and Italian bread, muffins, popovers, cornbread, baking powder biscuits, Zwieback, rusks, pretzels, matzoh, rolls, gluten bread, bagels, croutons, Sally Lunn, scones, doughnuts

Table 14. Elimination Diets

Diet One	Diet Two
Beverages	
Apricot juice	Apple juice
Lemonade	Grape juice
Pineapple juice	Prune juice
Tea	Coffee
	Milk
Cereal	
Pure corn	Rice
Hominy grits	
Meat	
Lamb, any cut	Beef, any cut
Pork, any cut	Chicken, any cut
(bacon, ham)	Veal, any cut
Vegetables	
Asparagus	Beets
Beans, all kinds	Carrots
Cabbage	Lettuce
Corn	Squash
Sweet potato	Turnips
Fruit	
Apricots	Apples
Banana	Grapes and raisins
Lemon	Plums
Pears	Prunes
Pineapple	
Bread	
Corn pone	100 percent rye bread and wafers
Fat	
Bacon fat	Butter
Mazola oil	Chicken fat

Table 14. (Continued)

Diet One	Diet Two
Miscellaneous	
Apricot jam	Apple butter
Gelatin	Apple jelly
Karo syrup	Cider vinegar
Molasses	Cheese
Salt	Gelatin
Sugar	Grape jelly
Synthetic vinegar	Salt
	Sugar

Cereals

Diet One	Diet Two
All Bran	Product 19
Apple Jacks	Protein Plus
Bran Flakes	Puffed Wheat
Cheerios	Raisin Bran
Cocoa Puffs	Ralston—regular, instant shredded
Crackles	Shredded Wheat
Cream of Wheat	Special K
Farina	Sugar Crisp
Froot Loops	Sugar Smacks
Grape-nuts	Total
Grape-nut Flakes	Trix
Infant type-mixed	Wheat Chex
Jets	Wheat Flakes
Kix	Wheat Honeys
Krumbles	Wheat germ
Maltex	Wheat Puffs
Maypo	Wheaties
Mellow Wheat	Wheatsworth
Muffets	Wheatena
Peps	Whole Bran
Pettijohn	

Flours

Wheat flour in any form including graham, white or whole wheat

Desserts

Cakes, cookies, doughnuts, pies, ice cream cones, pastries, puddings and prepared mixes except those especially made without wheat

Miscellaneous

Macaroni, spaghetti, noodles, vermicelli, pastina and other pasta
Dumplings, griddle cakes, waffles, pancakes, French toast, pizza, ravioli
Commercial candies that contain wheat
Gravies and sauces thickened with flour, commercial spaghetti and other sauces made with wheat
Soups containing wheat or wheat products, including canned broth or consomme
Fish or meats prepared with flour, bread or cracker crumbs, such as croquettes, meat loaf and stew thickened with flour
Commercially prepared meat, such as frankfurters, sausages and cold cuts where wheat may be used as a filler
Salad dressings—cooked or boiled—where flour is used for thickening

Acceptable bread and other baked products can be made with all soy, rice, corn or potato flour or cornmeal; 100 percent rye breads, crackers and wafers are available in some stores.

Egg-Free Diet

Omit these foods.

Bagels prepared with egg
Breads prepared with egg
Cake
Cookies
Crackers prepared with egg
Cream-type pies, such as lemon, custard, pumpkin, coconut, etc.
Custard
Doughnuts
Eclairs
Eggs
Eggnog or other egg drinks

Fish or meat prepared with egg, such as meat loaf, croquettes, breaded meats
Foods containing albumin
French toast
Fritters
Frosting prepared with egg
Griddle cakes
Hollandaise sauce
Ice cream
Macaroons
Marshmallows

Marshmallow Fluff
Mayonnaise and salad dressings
Meringue
Milk puddings containing eggs
Muffins
Noodles
Popovers
Pretzels
Ravioli
Soft candy, such as chocolate
    cream, nougat or fondant
Soft rolls prepared with egg
Sweet rolls and pastries
Rusks
Tartar sauce
Vaccines made in egg, such as
    influenza
Waffles
Yorkshire pudding and Zwieback

Milk-Free Diet

Omit any foods and commercial mixes containing milk, dried milk solids, casein, lactalbumin or curds and/or whey.

Bread made with milk
Butter and margarine (unless parve)
Cake, candies and cookies made
    with milk or milk products
Caramels
Cereals prepared with milk, such as
    Cocoa Krispies, Fortified Oat
    Flakes, Special K, Total
Cheese
Chocolate candy
Cocoa beverages
Cocomalt
Crackers made with milk
Cream
Cream or soft pies
Cream sauce
Cream soup
Creamed or scalloped foods
Custard
Doughnuts
Frosting prepared with milk
Gravies with milk and cream
Ice cream
Instant breakfast mixes
Instant cocoa mix
Malted milk
Milk
Milk, condensed
Milk, evaporated
Milk, powdered
Milk, skimmed
Milk puddings
Milk sherbets
Ovaltine
Potato mashed with milk
Pream

Rusks   Yogurt
Sweet rolls and pastries   Zwieback
Vegetables with milk or cream

This information is adapted from the Diet Manual of the Presbyterian Hospital in the City of New York at the Columbia-Presbyterian Medical Center.

Sources for Specific Diet Information

Allergy Information Association
25 Poynter Drive, Room 7
Weston, Ontario
M9R 1K8 Canada

American Allergy Association
P.O. Box 7273
Menlo Park, CA 94025

American Council on Science & Health
47 Maple Street
Summit, NJ 07901
Ask for "Food Additives and Hyperactivity"

American Dietetic Association
430 North Michigan Avenue
Chicago, IL 60611

Chicago Dietetic Supply, Inc.
405 East Shawmut Avenue
La Grange, IL 60525
A source for many products used in various allergy diets.

Ener-G Foods, Inc.
6901 Fox Avenue South
P.O. Box 24723
Seattle, WA
Recipes for gluten-free, milk-free, wheat-free, soy-free, corn-free, and no-added-preservatives diets are available. This company is also a source for a variety of foods used for specialized diets.

General Foods Consumer Center
Nutrition Services
250 North Street
White Plains, NY 10625
Ask for "Special Recipes & Allergy Aids"

Good Housekeeping Bulletin Service
959 8th Avenue
New York, NY 10019
Ask for "125 Great Recipes for Allergy Diets"

Human Nutrition Center
U.S. Dept. of Agriculture
14th Street and Independence Avenue SW
Washington, DC 20850

Loma Linda Foods
11503 Pierce Street
Riverside, CA 92515
Ask for "Delicious Milk-Free Recipes"

Mead Johnson & Company
Nutritional Division
Evansville, IN 47721
Ask for "Meals Without Milk"

National Celiac-Sprye Society
5 Jeffrey Road
Wayland, MA 01778
Ask for "Gluten-Free Diet"

Rice Council of America
P.O. Box 74021
Houston, TX 77274
Ask for "Tasty Rice Recipes for Those with Allergies"

Environmental Control Products and Sources

Air Filtering Devices

Contact local heating and air conditioning contractors to get additional information regarding electronic air purifiers. Units may be used for a single room or centrally installed with a compatible heating system.

Cleanaire HEPA
Bio-Tech Systems
P.O. Box 25380
Chicago, IL 60625

Hepanaire Air Cleaner
Summit Hill Laboratories
429 Highway 36
P.O. Box 535
Navesink, NJ 07752

Honeywell Clean Air Machine
Honeywell Plaza
Minneapolis, MN 55408

Space-Gard Air Cleaner
Research Products Corporation
P.O. Box 1467
Madison, WI 53701

Humidifiers   The most efficient types of individual room humidifiers are of the ultrasonic variety. These units are currently produced by most of the major appliance companies in the country. These units are highly efficient and run silently.

Dehumidifiers   In highly damp environments dehumidifiers can be very effective in decreasing the growth of molds. Molds are a major source of trouble for many allergic children.

The following companies sell their dehumidifiers nationally: Fedders, Kelvinator, Oasis and Comfort Air.

Dust and Mold Control

These companies provide dust covers for mattresses, box springs and pillows. Mold- and dust-control preparations are also available from them.

Allergen-Proof Encasing
1450 East 363rd Street
Eastlake, OH 44094

Allergy Control Products
28 High Ridge Road
Ridgefield, CT 06877

Bio-Tech Systems
P.O. Box 25380
Chicago, IL 60625

Environment Corporation
P.O. Box 31313
St. Louis, MO 63131

Allergy Organizations

National

Asthma & Allergy Foundation of America
1302 18th Street N.W.
Suite 303
Washington, DC 20036
(202) 293-2950

American Association of Certified Allergists
401 East Prospect Avenue Suite 210
Mount Prospect, IL 60056
(312) 255-1024

American College of Allergists
800 East Northwest Highway
Suite 101
Mount Prospect, IL 60056
(312) 255-0380

National Institute of Allergy and Infectious Diseases
9000 Rockville Pike
Bethesda, MD 20205
(301) 496-2263

American Association for Clinical Immunology and Allergy
P.O. Box 912
Omaha, NE 68101
(402) 551-0801

American Academy of Allergy and Immunology
611 East Wells Street
Milwaukee, WI 53202
(414) 272-6071

Pulmonary (Lung) Organizations

American Lung Association
1740 Broadway
New York, NY 10019
(212) 245-8000

American Thoracic Society
1740 Broadway

New York, NY 10019
(212) 245-8000

National Heart, Lung and Blood Institute
NIH
Bethesda, MD 20205

Major Research Centers of Immunological Diseases

UCLA School of Medicine
Center for Health Sciences Building
Los Angeles, CA 90024

Georgetown University School of Medicine
3900 Reservoir Road, NW
Washington, DC 20007

Children's Hospital Medical Center
300 Longwood Avenue
Boston, MA 02115

The Johns Hopkins University School of Medicine
Good Samaritan Hospital
5601 Loch Raven Boulevard
Baltimore, MD 21239

Washington University School of Medicine
660 South Euclid Avenue
St. Louis, MO 63110

University of Rochester
School of Medicine and Dentistry
601 Elmwood Avenue
Rochester, NY 14642

Asthma and Allergy Diseases Centers

Scripps Clinic and Research
  Foundation
10666 North Torrey Pines Road
La Jolla, CA 92037

University of California-San Diego
  Medical Center
255 Dickinson Center
San Diego, CA 92103

University of California-San
  Francisco
Department of Medicine
400 Parnassus Avenue
San Francisco, CA 94143

Northwestern University Medical
  School
303 East Chicago Avenue
Chicago, IL 60611

University of Iowa Hospitals
Department of Internal Medicine
Division of Allergy and
  Immunology
Iowa City, IA 52242

Tulane University School of
  Medicine
1700 Perdido Street
New Orleans, LA 70112

National Institutes of Health,
  NIAID
Building 10, Room 11N250
Bethesda, MD 20205

Harvard Medical School
75 Francis Street
Boston, MA 02111

Tufts University School of Medicine
136 Harrison Avenue
Boston, MA 02111

The Rockefeller University
1230 York Avenue
New York, NY 10021

State University of NY at Stony
    Brook
Health Sciences Center
Stony Brook, NY 11794

Duke University
P.O. Box 2893
Durham, NC 27710

University of Texas Health Sciences
    Center
Dermatology Division
5223 Harry Hynes Boulevard
Dallas, TX 75235

Medical College of Wisconsin
Department of Medicine
8700 West Wisconsin Avenue
P.O. Box 12
Milwaukee, WI 53226

Glossary

Words set in small caps are defined elsewhere in the Glossary.

ADRENALIN. *See* EPINEPHRINE

AIR POLLUTION.   A major problem in most industrial and urban areas of the United States, and an aggravating factor for those who suffer from respiratory allergies. Compounds such as sulfur dioxide and carbon monoxide are two of the many chemical substances that can precipitate asthma attacks in susceptible individuals.

ALLERGENIC.   Capable of causing an allergic reaction.

ALLERGENIC EXTRACT.   Substance employed in the diagnosis and treatment of allergic individuals. The most commonly used of these are water-based substances known as aqueous extracts. They are prepared by grinding and removing the fat from the original material, placing the allergenic portion of the material into an extraction fluid (most often a buffered saltwater solution), passing the material through a glass column (dialyzing column), and sterilizing the final product; it is then ready for use as a diagnostic and therapeutic agent. A long-standing problem with allergenic extracts has been standardization: how to guarantee that one hundred units of company A's product—say, ragweed extract—is equal to one hundred units of company B's product. This dilemma, as yet unresolved, can under certain conditions complicate the treatment of a patient who moves from one part of the country to another or who switches from one doctor to another.

A number of allergenic extracts will soon be commercially available which are chemically processed in such a way that fewer injections will be required in order for a patient to reach a maintenance dose. These injections will be given at less frequent intervals than those which come in aqueous extracts. They are called polymerized allergens.

ALLERGEN.   Special type of ANTIGEN, i.e., any substance foreign to the human body, capable of triggering allergic symptoms in a sensitized person.

279

Exposure to an allergen may come through contact with the skin, from ingestion, or from inhalation. Common allergens include mold spores, pollen grains
from trees, grasses and weeds, dust, mites, danders, feathers, moldspores and
industrial and occupational dust, substances. *See* ANTIGEN

ALLERGIC IgE ANTIBODY. An ANTIBODY that, when interacting with a
specific ANTIGEN, is responsible for producing allergic reactions. For example,
in order to develop symptoms of hay fever a person's body must first produce
antiragweed IgE antibodies and then be exposed to the ragweed pollen. The
reaction of these two substances will combine to cause the sneezing, tearing
eyes and runny nose typical of hay fever. The human body is capable of
producing multimillions of different antibodies; while most of us produce small
amounts of IgE, allergic individuals have high levels in their bloodstream. The
IgE level is a general indicator of a person's potential for developing allergic
symptoms.

ALLERGIC BRONCHOPULMONARY ASPERGILLOSIS. An unusual lung ailment
which sometimes occurs in patients suffering from allergic asthma. The condition is caused by infection with a fungus called aspergillus.

ALLERGIC RHINITIS. A complex of symptoms consisting of sneeze, runny
nose, and itchy nose which may occur as a seasonal problem, called rose fever
or hay fever, or as a year-round condition known as perennial allergic rhinitis.

ALLERGIC SHINERS. Dark circles which form under the eyes, commonly seen
in allergic children, caused by local swelling and a sluggish blood flow throughout the many capillary blood vessels surrounding the eyes.

ALLERGIST. A physician who has gone through at least a two-year period of
specialized training in the diagnosis and treatment of allergic diseases. A
doctor must be eligible to take the certifying examination or must be certified
by the board of allergy and immunology in order to be recognized as a
specialist in allergic diseases.

ALLERGOID. An ALLERGENIC substance that has been chemically modified
so that its ability to produce allergic reactions is significantly decreased but its
capacity to stimulate protective IgG antibody production remains unchanged.
These materials are being studied today for possible use as immunizing agents
for allergic patients.

ALLERGY. A pathological reaction to environmental substances such as
foods, pollens, dust and so on. The term was derived from the Greek words
allos (other) and *ergeon* (action). People who suffer from allergies develop an

"altered response" when exposed to specific environmental substances. This response is both protective (as an immune response) and harmful (it can cause a person to become hypersensitive). In common usage the term *allergy* has become synonymous with hypersensitivity.

ALVEOLI. The small, balloonlike air sacs located at the ends of the smallest air passageways in the lungs. Oxygen and carbon dioxide transfer takes place in the alveoli.

AMINOPHYLLINE. A form of THEOPHYLLINE used in the treatment of bronchial asthma.

ANAPHYLACTOID. A generalized reaction that mimics an anaphylactic response but that is not caused by an allergic, IgE-mediated reaction. A common example is the response certain patients experience when injected with contrast media for X-ray studies, especially the media used for an intravenous pyelogram. *See* ANAPHYLAXIS

ANAPHYLAXIS. A term used to define a severe, GENERALIZED ALLERGIC REACTION occurring either immediately or several hours after exposure to an ALLERGEN. Symptoms may include local or generalized hives or ANGIO-EDEMA, persistent sneezing, continuous watery nasal discharge, shortness of breath, tightness in the chest, wheezing, swelling of the throat and larynx, a drop in blood pressure, unconsciousness and possibly death. These symptoms take place following the massive release of a variety of chemical substances, called MEDIATORS.

ANGIOEDEMA. A localized swelling in the deeper layers of the skin generally caused by an allergic reaction. There is rarely any itching associated with angioedema. While typical areas of swelling include the lips, eyelids, feet and hands, angioedema can occur in virtually any part of the body. *See* URTICARIA

ANTIBODY. A special type of protein manufactured by plasma cells in response to any foreign substance (or ANTIGEN) entering the body. Once produced, the antibody is capable of reacting only with its specific antigen. For example, in order to become sensitized to a cat, a dog or tree pollen, a child's body must first produce specific antibodies against cat, dog or tree antigens.

Allergic antibodies are collectively found in a class of proteins called IgE. There are also other antibody types, a majority of them involved in the body's defense mechanism against infection. Most common of these is gammaglobulin or IgG. Other antibody groups are labeled IgA, IgM and IgD. *See* IMMUNO-GLOBULIN

ANTIGEN.   Any foreign substance that causes specific antibodies to be produced in the body and which has the capacity to stimulate an immune response. For example, exposure to dog antigen in a child may cause the production of antidog IgE antibodies in that child. During a lifetime the body is exposed to millions and millions of antigens. It responds by producing a specific antibody for each. *See* ANTIBODY

ANTIHISTAMINE.   A family of drugs used in the treatment of common allergic symptoms such as sneezing, runny nose, tearing eyes and itching. The many antihistamines on the market today come from five distinct chemical groups plus a sixth group labeled miscellaneous. Antihistamines work by blocking the effect of the chemical substance histamine, which is manufactured and released by the body during an allergic reaction. *See* HISTAMINE

ANTISERUM.   An immunizing agent which contains antibodies and which is used to prevent certain infections. For example, an antiserum prepared for use against tetanus contains a protective ANTIBODY against specific tetanus toxins. (When used against a toxin an antiserum is known as an antitoxin.)

One traditional method of producing tetanus antitoxin is to immunize an animal such as a horse with tetanus germs and then collect the antibodies from the horse's blood. The horse serum containing the protective antibodies is then injected into a human being who is at risk of developing tetanus. While at one time antiserum made from horses was quite commonly used against tetanus, the pharmaceutical industry today markets a tetanus antitoxin, known as Hypertet, derived almost exclusively from human beings.

ARTERIAL BLOOD GAS DETERMINATION.   The respiratory gases oxygen and carbon dioxide are normally found in the bloodstream. During a severe or prolonged asthma attack, important changes take place in the amounts of these gases in the body. In order to appropriately treat the asthmatic patient, a specimen of arterial blood is analyzed for its blood gas concentration.

ASTHMA.   A condition characterized by reversible episodes of airway obstruction which range in severity from mild to life threatening. Common symptoms include shortness of breath, chest tightness, coughing and wheezing. Children do not have to be allergic to have asthma, though they often are. Asthma can be broadly divided into three forms: allergic or extrinsic immunologic, nonallergic or intrinsic/autonomic, and mixed.

ATOPIC DERMATITIS.   A form of eczema, an allergic skin condition characterized by dry skin and a very itchy rash, commonly located on the cheeks, backs of the ears, elbows, wrists and backs of the knees.

ATOPY.   The state or condition of being allergic.

AUTOGENOUS. Self-generated. In allergic medicine, most commonly used to describe a vaccine prepared from bacteria taken directly from a patient's body.

B CELLS. One of two special types of white blood cells called lymphocytes produced in the bone marrow. *See* LYMPHOCYTE

BACTERIAL VACCINES. Vaccines prepared from common bacteria. For example, streptococcus and staphylococcus vaccines are used in the treatment of so-called bacterial allergy.

At best the use of these vaccines must be considered controversial; and while we know that viral infections can play a definite role in triggering attacks of bronchial asthma, no sound evidence exists proving that a person can become truly allergic to a specific bacteria. There is general agreement among experts that there is no use for bacterial vaccines in the treatment of allergic diseases.

BACTERIAL ALLERGY. *See* BACTERIAL VACCINES

BASOPHIL. A specific type of white blood cell that circulates freely throughout the bloodstream and which is coated with IgE antibodies. When this cell is stimulated to release chemical MEDIATORS, an allergic reaction is set in motion. *See* MEDIATOR

BETA-ADRENERGIC AGENT. *See* BRONCHODILATOR

BLOOD GASES. Gases, such as oxygen and carbon dioxide, in constant circulation throughout the bloodstream. During a severe asthma attack insufficient amounts of oxygen reach the blood and increased levels of carbon dioxide accumulate.

BRONCHIAL CHALLENGE TEST. Inhaling an aerosolized spray containing an ALLERGEN suspected of causing asthma. This procedure should be done under the direct supervision of a doctor, in a laboratory setting. The test can also be done using the drugs histamine or methacholine.

BRONCHODILATOR DRUG. A drug that causes the bronchial tubes to relax and dilate, commonly used in the treatment of bronchial asthma, some forms of chronic bronchitis, and occasionally in adults suffering from emphysema. The two main types of bronchodilator drugs are methylxanthines such as THEOPHYLLINE and BETA-ADRENERGIC AGENTS such as metaproterenol.

BRONCHOSPASM. Constriction or narrowing of the bronchial air passageways that causes wheezing.

CHALLENGE TESTING.   *See* BRONCHIAL CHALLENGE TEST, NASAL CHALLENGE TEST, ORAL CHALLENGE TEST

CBC.   Complete blood count, a blood test used to check the number of red blood cells, white blood cells and amount of hemoglobin in a patient's body and to study specific types of circulating white blood cells (a differential count) to determine the presence of infection, anemia or allergy.

CLINICAL ECOLOGY.   A controversial new area of medical practice in which a variety of vague, fairly common symptoms not generally felt to be allergic are attributed to an undiagnosed and unrecognized allergy. A number of the diagnostic and therapeutic procedures used by clinical ecologists have been found to be both unreliable and ineffective. There is presently no valid scientific evidence supporting the medical claims of this "specialty" in regards to many of its methods of diagnosis and treatment.

CONTACT DERMATITIS.   An allergic rash that appears after exposure to a plant, chemical or metallic object to which a person has become sensitized. Inflammation is always localized in the area of specific contact. Common examples include poison ivy, skin reactions to cosmetics or detergents and sensitivity to the nickel found in jewelry.

CORTICOSTEROIDS.   A group of naturally occurring hormones and commercially prepared agents which are powerful anti-inflammatory and antiallergic drugs. Cortisone, produced naturally by the adrenal glands and manufactured commercially by pharmaceutical companies, is the best known of this rather large family. Many side effects are associated with them, one of the most common being weight gain. Use of corticosteroids must *always* be closely supervised by a physician.

CROMOLYN SODIUM.   The generic name for a drug used to treat asthma (in the form of Intal), allergic rhinitis (as Nasalcrom) and allergic conjunctivitis (as Opticrom). Unlike BRONCHODILATOR DRUGS, which actively dilate the bronchial airways during an asthma attack, cromolyn has the ability to prevent the symptoms of asthma from developing. Cromolyn has an extremely low incidence of side effects, which makes it especially safe for children.

CYTOTOXIC TESTING.   An unproven diagnostic test used for evaluating food allergies, which does *not* work. The Food and Drug Administration (FDA) has labeled this procedure "unreliable as a diagnostic test."

DANDERS.   The dead superficial layers of skin that flake off an animal, producing allergic symptoms in a sensitized person.

DECONGESTANTS. Drugs used mainly for the control of nasal symptoms associated with the common cold, allergic rhinitis (hay fever) and vasomotor rhinitis. Both spray and drop forms should never be taken for more than five days in a row; if used for longer periods they may not only lose their effectiveness but will actually cause nasal congestion.

DERMATOGRAPHISM. A congenital condition in which the skin has a high degree of irritability. A raised wheal and redness appear on the skin when it is stroked or rubbed with a blunt object. Because of this nonspecific response pattern, a child with dermatographism is not a satisfactory candidate for direct skin tests (scratch or prick/puncture). *See* RAST TEST

DESENSITIZATION. *See* IMMUNOTHERAPY

DIRECT SKIN TEST. The simplest and most sensitive method to detect the presence of allergic IgE ANTIBODIES. *See* INTRADERMAL TEST, PRICK/PUNCTURE TEST, SCRATCH TEST

DUST MITES Microscopic insects that live mainly in bed linens and which are thought by some investigators to be the main allergen found in dust.

ECZEMA. A condition of the skin characterized by a rash that is extremely itchy, scaly and dry. *See* ATOPIC DERMATITIS, CONTACT DERMATITIS

ECZEMATOUS. Characteristic of a condition of ECZEMA.

ELIMINATION DIET. A procedure whereby a certain food is eliminated from a patient's diet for a trial period and the patient's reaction observed. If the symptoms disappear, the food is reintroduced to see if the symptoms return. This procedure must be repeated twice before a definite relationship is proven between the specific food and the allergy symptom.

EMPHYSEMA A chronic lung disease, limited almost exclusively to adults, that causes destruction of the ALVEOLI. Rarely if ever is there any relationship between asthma and emphysema. Damage to the lungs in emphysema is permanent and the changes are irreversible.

ENVIRONMENTAL CONTROL. With IMMUNOTHERAPY and pharmacotherapy, one of the three major methods of managing allergic conditions.

EOSINOPHIL. A type of white blood cell of which allergic patients usually show an increased number in their bloodstream, determined by a differential white blood cell count.

EPINEPHRINE. A chemical produced by the human adrenal glands and frequently used to treat bronchial asthma and allergic emergencies. Available as Adrenalin or the long-acting form, Sus-Phrine.

ERYTHROCYTE SEDIMENTATION RATE (ESR). A blood test, taken by VENIPUNCTURE, which indicates whether an inflammation (infection) is present somewhere within a patient's body. If the ESR value is positive, then other more specific diagnostic tests must be performed.

EXERCISE-INDUCED ASTHMA (EIA). A condition in which wheezing occurs after a period of strenuous physical activity; most common during the colder months of the year, especially following outdoor exertion, it occurs in 70 to 80 percent of all asthma patients.

FUNGI. *See* MOLDS

GASTROESOPHAGEAL REFUX REFLEX (GER). A condition that occurs due to an improperly functioning gastroesophageal sphincter muscle, which permits the backup of stomach fluids into the esophagus. Associated with recurrent cough and wheezing in infancy, a number of tests exist to diagnosis it. These include X-ray studies, barium swallow, checking the acid level of the esophagus fluid (pH monitoring), and pressure studies (manometry). Treatment involves thickened feedings, propping the infant up in an upright position after meals, and possibly surgery to repair the esophageal sphincter, if medical treatment fails.

GENERALIZED ALLERGIC REACTION. A reaction involving several organ systems at once. May involve the lungs (wheezing), the skin (hives), the nose and eyes (sneezing and tearing), and the cardiovascular system (rapid heartbeat, drop in blood pressure). *See* ANAPHYLAXIS

HAY FEVER. A common term for a pattern of symptoms that occur during the pollinating seasons of trees, grasses and weeds, and which is medically known as seasonal RHINITIS. Symptoms may include a runny nose, sneezing, tearing, itchy eyes, nasal congestion, fatigue and irritability. There is no fever involved with hay fever, nor is it caused by hay.

HISTAMINE. The cause of the itching, runny nose, teary eyes and swelling typically associated with hay fever and eczema. *See* MEDIATOR.

HIVES. *See* URTICARIA

HOUSE DUST. Dust composed of the breakdown products of organic fibers such as wool and cotton as well as animal danders, insect residues, bacteria, food substances, mold spores and so on. *See* DUST MITES

HYMENOPTERA.   An order of insects responsible for the majority of allergic sting reactions. Members include bees, wasps, hornets, yellow jackets and fire ants.

HYPERSENSITIVITY.   A state of the immune system in which harmful symptoms are produced in the individual, as opposed to the normally beneficial responses of the immune system. There are four major types of hypersensitivity response: ANAPHYLACTIC, cytotoxic, immune complex mediated and cell mediated or delayed.

HYPOALLERGENIC.   A term referring to substances which have a very low potential to sensitize people or to cause an allergic reaction.

HYPOSENSITIZATION.   *See* IMMUNOTHERAPY

IMMEDIATE HYPERSENSITIVITY.   An allergic reaction involving the IgE class of immunoglobulin proteins, also referred to as anaphylactic hypersensitivity. Examples include allergic rhinitis, penicillin allergy, allergic asthma and anaphylactic shock.

IMMUNE SYSTEM.   The physiological system that guards and protects the body against bacteria, viruses, cancer cells, chemicals and, under certain unusual conditions, one's own organs. The immune system includes the thymus gland, the bone marrow, the lymph nodes (glands), the spleen and specialized lymph tissues in the intestinal tract. A number of different types of cells play a crucial role in this system. These include white blood cells called LYMPHOCYTES, EOSINOPHILS, and monocyte-macrophages. Without a properly functioning immune system, humans could not survive.

IMMUNOGLOBULINS.   Special type of protein produced by the body. There are five classes of immunoglobulins (Ig), designated IgM, IgA, IgD, IgG and IgE. The IgM, IgA and IgG classes are responsible for protecting the body against invasion by viruses and bacteria. The function of IgD is still unclear. IgE antibodies are involved primarily with allergic reactions.

The various immunoglobulins are produced by a special type of lymphocyte (a white blood cell) called a plasma cell.

IMMUNOTHERAPY.   A form of allergy treatment commonly referred to as "desensitization," hyposensitization or "allergy shots." Treatment consists of increasing a patient's tolerance to an allergenic substance by means of a graduated program of injections that contain ever-increasing doses of the allergen. The average length of treatment can be anywhere from two to four years. When successful, immunotherapy will reduce the intensity and duration of clinical allergic symptoms, though it will not necessarily eliminate them completely. Recommended for allergic rhinitis, severe insect sting sensitivity and allergic asthma.

INTRADERMAL TEST.   The most sensitive form of direct skin test available in which a small amount of allergen is injected by a needle or syringe into the superficial layers of the skin.

IN VITRO TEST.   A test done in the laboratory.

IN VIVO TEST.   A test done directly on the patient.

KAPOK.   A fiber derived from the kapok tree, commonly used as a filler for decorative pillows and as a stuffing for upholstered furniture. It is a common allergen.

LACTOSE INTOLERANCE.   A condition arising from the absence of an enzyme called lactase in the small intestine and generally characterized by chronic diarrhea. Often seen in infants, its symptoms begin shortly after the introduction of either human or cow's milk to the diet and tend to clear up immediately if a nonmilk formula such as a soybean preparation is substituted. Lactose intolerance is usually a lifelong condition, and sufferers must make all efforts to avoid all sources of milk such as milk, cheese, cream and so on. This is not an allergic condition but rather an enzyme deficiency disease.

LUNG FUNCTION TEST.   *See* PULMONARY FUNCTION TEST

LYMPHOCYTE.   A type of white blood cell that plays an important role in the immune process. In one of its specialized forms, as a plasma cell it is responsible for producing ANTIBODIES. Classified into two groups: the T cell lymphocyte that originates in the thymus gland and the B cell lymphocyte that comes from bone marrow. A complicated relationship exists between the B and T lymphocytes as they work together in many types of immune responses.

MAST CELL.   A cell found in body tissues, that is coated with IgE antibodies in allergic individuals. When these antibodies react with their specific antigens, an allergic reaction takes place, the end result being the release of a number of chemical MEDIATORS (such as HISTAMINE or SRS-A) with the consequent development of allergic symptoms.

MEDIATOR.   A chemical compound released from the basophil and mast cells during an allergic reaction. Sneezing, tearing eyes, a watery, drippy nose and wheezing are the most typical allergic symptoms caused by the various chemical mediators. *See* HISTAMINE, SRS-A

MOLDS.   Plants that do not possess chlorophyll and which therefore depend on outside sources of nourishment. Over 75,000 different varieties have been identified, many of which may cause allergic symptoms. *See* SPORES

MUCUS.   The viscous fluid secreted by the mucus glands to moisten and protect the MUCOUS MEMBRANES. Mucus varies in consistency from a thin, watery secretion to a thick, yellow-green discharge. Mucus-secreting glands line the respiratory tract from the nose to the smallest airways of the lungs.

MUCOUS MEMBRANES.   The linings of the mouth, throat, nose and respiratory system.

NASAL CHALLENGE TEST.   This is a test in which a suspension containing a suspected ALLERGEN is sprayed into the nose in order to determine if the person is allergic. The procedure should always be done in a laboratory setting, supervised by a physician.

NASAL POLYPS.   Round, soft, jellylike masses found in the sinuses and nasal passageways. Most commonly clear to whitish in color, they may grow individually or in grape-like clusters. In childhood they are most commonly associated with cystic fibrosis. While severely allergic children can under certain conditions develop polyps, they are more commonly found in adults. Treatment for polyps requires the use of topical cortisone sprays as a shrinking agent. If this measure fails, surgical removal is often the only alternative; unfortunately there is a high rate of regrowth of surgically removed polyps.

ORAL CHALLENGE TEST.   Eating a food containing a suspected ALLERGEN to determine if an allergy is present; always done under the direct supervision of a doctor.

OTITIS MEDIA.   An inflammation of the middle ear especially common in young children.

PATCH TEST.   A method used to identify substances responsible for causing allergic responses, specifically CONTACT DERMATITIS. The suspected material is placed on a small area of the skin, usually on the arm or back, and covered with an adhesive patch. After forty-eight hours the test site is checked. The presence of an itchy, blistery area is considered to be a positive response, indicating that the person is allergic to the test substance.

PENICILLIN ALLERGY.   One of the most common types of drug allergy, the symptoms of which can range from a mild skin rash to a life-threatening, generalized ANAPHYLACTIC response. A method of testing for this allergy exists but can only identify a person who is allergic to penicillin after the individual has displayed some symptoms.

POLLEN.   A grain containing the male reproductive portion of trees, grasses and weeds. Microscopically small, it is carried long distances by the wind.

Allergy to the pollen is responsible for the symptoms of such conditions as allergic rhinitis and asthma.

PRICK TEST.   A form of direct skin test in which a drop of allergen is placed on the arm or back and the point of a needle is used to puncture the skin so that the allergen is able to react with the tissue mast cells.

PROVOCATIVE TESTING.   A procedure exposing patients to a specific allergen to determine if they are allergic to it. *See* BRONCHIAL CHALLENGE TEST, NASAL CHALLENGE TEST, ORAL CHALLENGE TEST

PRURITUS.   The medical term for itching.

PULMONARY FUNCTION TEST.   A test designed to obtain specific information indicating how efficiently a patient's lungs are operating.

RAST (RADIOALLERGOSORBENT TEST).   An in vitro method of allergy testing in which blood serum is examined and analyzed. Though generally reliable, it is less sensitive than certain forms of direct skin testing such as the INTRADERMAL TEST. It is also expensive and requires a good deal of time before the results are known. When direct skin tests cannot be performed, the RAST test is an acceptable alternative.

REAGINIC ANTIBODIES.   A term that refers to allergic antibodies of the IgE class of IMMUNOGLOBULINS.

REBOUND PHENOMENON.   A response to a medicine in which clinical symptoms worsen after the medication is discontinued.

RHINITIS   A nasal condition characterized by sneezing, nasal congestion and an increase in nasal discharge. Rhinitis can occur on a seasonal basis (when it is known as hay fever or rose fever), or it may be year-round as in perennial allergic rhinitis. *See* VASOMOTOR RHINITIS

RHINITIS MEDICAMENTOSA.   A condition that develops owing to prolonged use of vasoconstrictor nose drops or sprays.

RINKEL METHOD.   A controversial and unproven technique of immunotherapy using a graduated testing schedule; the purpose of this method is to determine both the appropriate starting dose and the so-called end point of therapy. Controlled studies have proven, however, that the end point dose is simply too low to produce a maximal response.

SCRATCH TEST. A procedure administered by placing a drop of ALLERGEN on the arm or back. A superficial scratch is made over the test site with the tip of a needle so that the allergen is absorbed directly into the skin.

SENSITIZED. Any person who has been exposed to an antigen (a foreign substance) that has stimulated the immune system to produce specific antibodies has become sensitized. For example, the hay fever sufferer has been sensitized to ragweed pollen.

SERUM. The clear, yellowish liquid portion of the blood that remains after a clot has formed and the white and red blood cells have settled out.

SHOCK ORGAN. The part of the body that is the site of an allergic reaction. The shock organ for allergic rhinitis is the nose; for bronchial asthma it is the lungs.

SRS-A. An abbreviation for slow-reacting substance of anaphylaxis, a powerful bronchoconstrictor MEDIATOR that is probably responsible for the severe prolonged bronchospasm which occurs during an asthma attack. Now known as leukotrienes.

STATUS ASTHMATICUS. A term describing an asthma attack so severe that it does not respond to oral and inhaled BRONCHODILATOR DRUGS. Patients who fail to respond to two or three injections of ADRENALIN given at twenty- to thirty-minute intervals are in status asthmaticus and will require hospitalization for more intensive treatment, which will usually include the administration of intravenous fluids, oxygen and cortisone.

STEROIDS. *See* CORTICOSTEROIDS

SPORES. Parts of the mold plant which contain the reproductive system. Microscopic in size, they float in the air and are found in profusion during spring, summer and early fall; a primary allergen for many allergy sufferers.

THEOPHYLLINE The most frequently prescribed BRONCHODILATOR DRUG in the United States, it exists in many different forms and brands and is especially effective against asthma.

TYMPANOMETRY. A sensitive procedure used to check for abnormalities of the tympanic membrane/middle ear/eustachian tube system and to evaluate middle ear function, it is painless and can be done in an office setting with children as young as seven months.

URTICARIA. A localized swelling in the superficial layers of the skin, commonly known as hives, the typical rash consists of red or white raised lesions surrounded by a reddish border; it can be recognized most directly by its severe, persistent itching. *See* ANGIOEDEMA.

VASOMOTOR RHINITIS.   A nasal condition characterized by symptoms which closely mimic those of HAY FEVER: nasal congestion, sneezing and (occasionally) a year-round runny nose; it occurs as a result of a nonspecific irritative response to a variety of *nonallergic* stimuli and is localized to the mucous membranes of the nose. This condition tends to become chronic, and treatment is geared toward controlling symptoms; so far no permanent cure exists.

VENOMS.   *See* HYMENOPTERA

WHEEZE.   The typical rattling, whistling, breathing sounds an asthmatic child makes when exhaling, primarily owing to the narrowing of the breathing tubes and the accumulation of thick mucus secretions within the air passageways.

Index

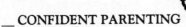